Much love to my two wonderful children who have been my greatest inspiration. You are the color of my life!

Thank you to each of you for drawing 2 images for me!!!!

Coloring a Mindful Journey
Artistically Express Yourself Through Color

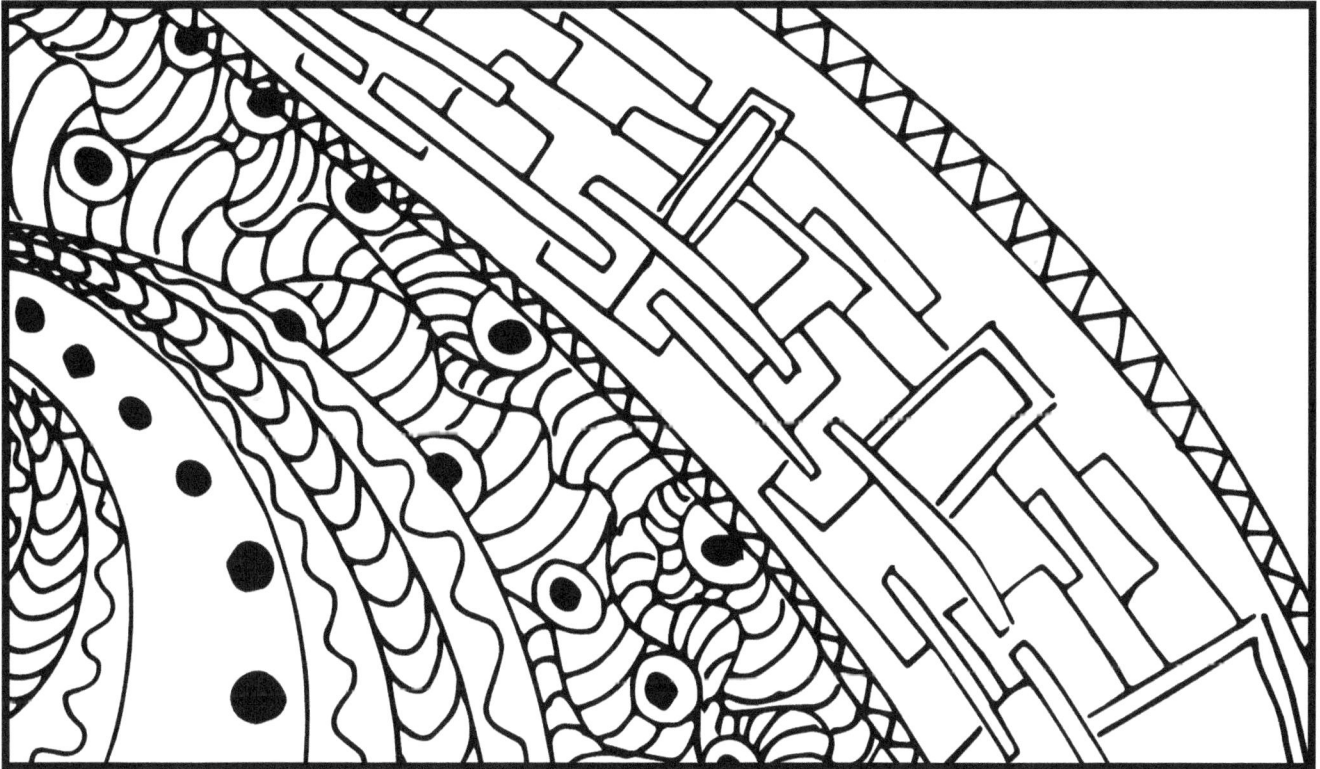

Sasha Scully is a professional artist who specializes in oil paintings, digital art, graphic design, teaching art, and using art and color as a tool for relaxation and self-discovery. With a rich background in the arts and engineering, she has shown her artwork in many different galleries and exhibits, juried art shows, been featured in several publications, and crafted award-winning art pieces.

As a mother of two and a professional artist living in New Mexico, she strives to create emotions through her work. She encourages others to do the same and create their own visual journeys through life. She uses painting, drawing, and coloring as a safe outlet for her feelings. Coloring and art is about how you feel with-in while you are creating. Embrace your feelings and enjoy living in the moment.

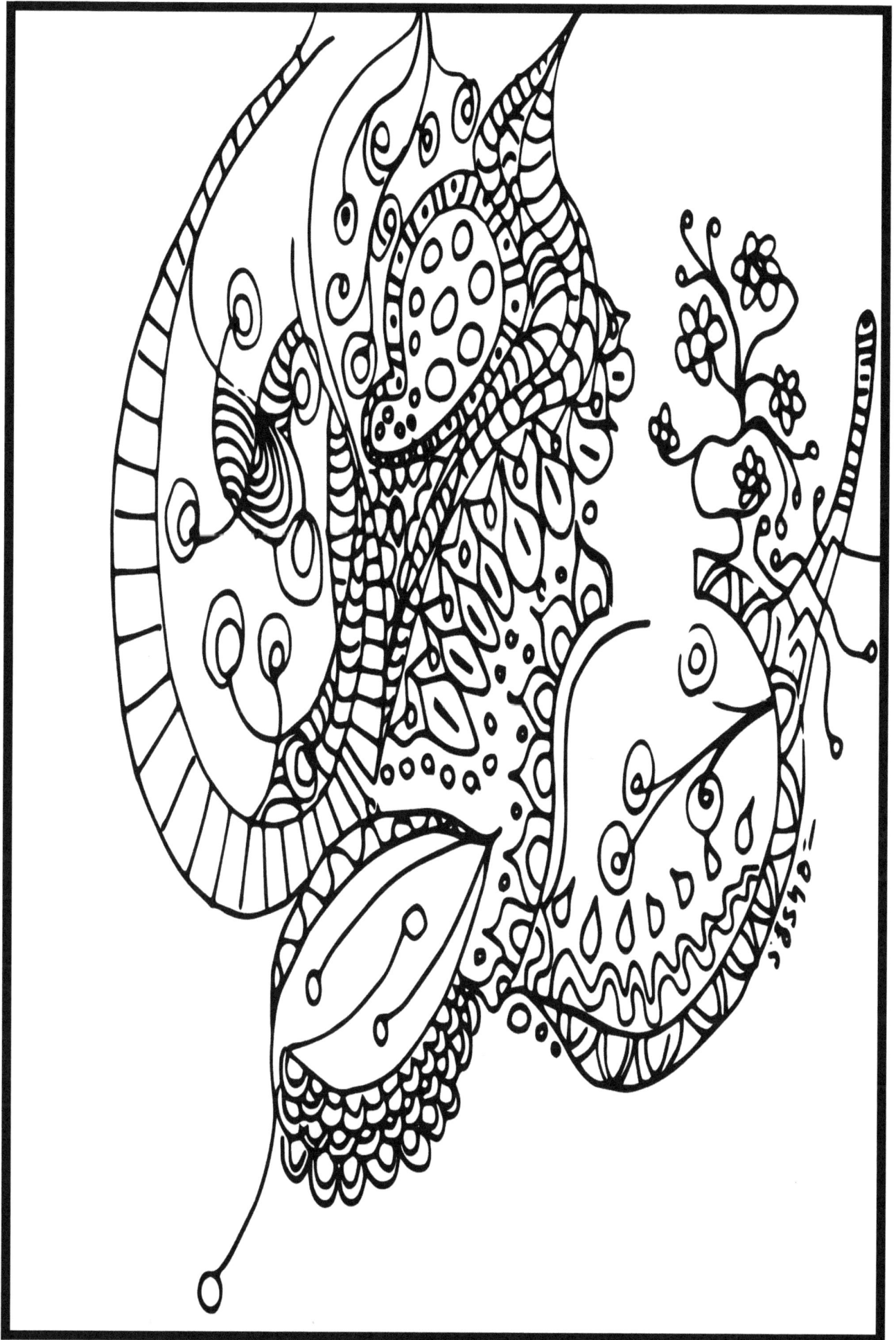

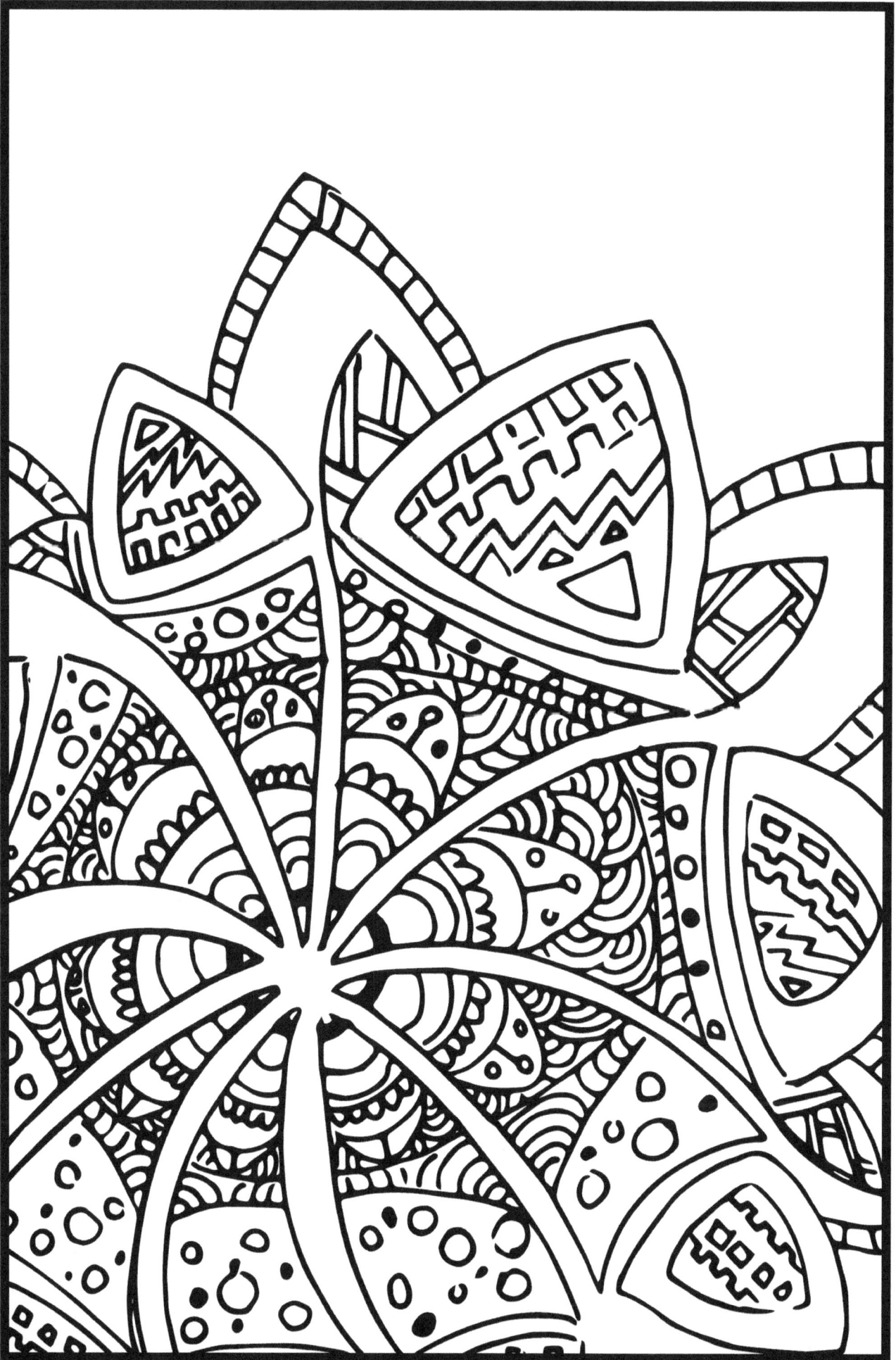

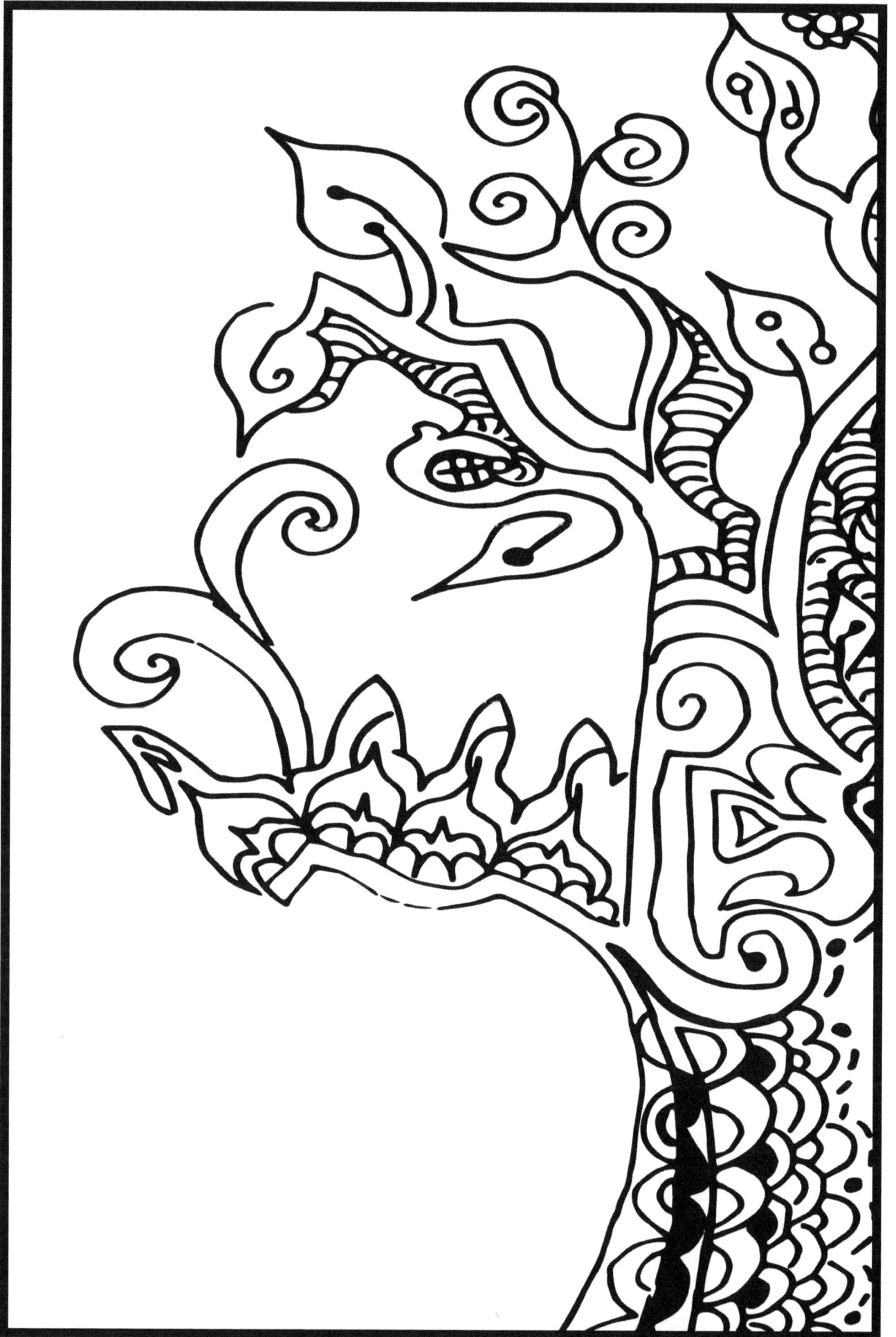

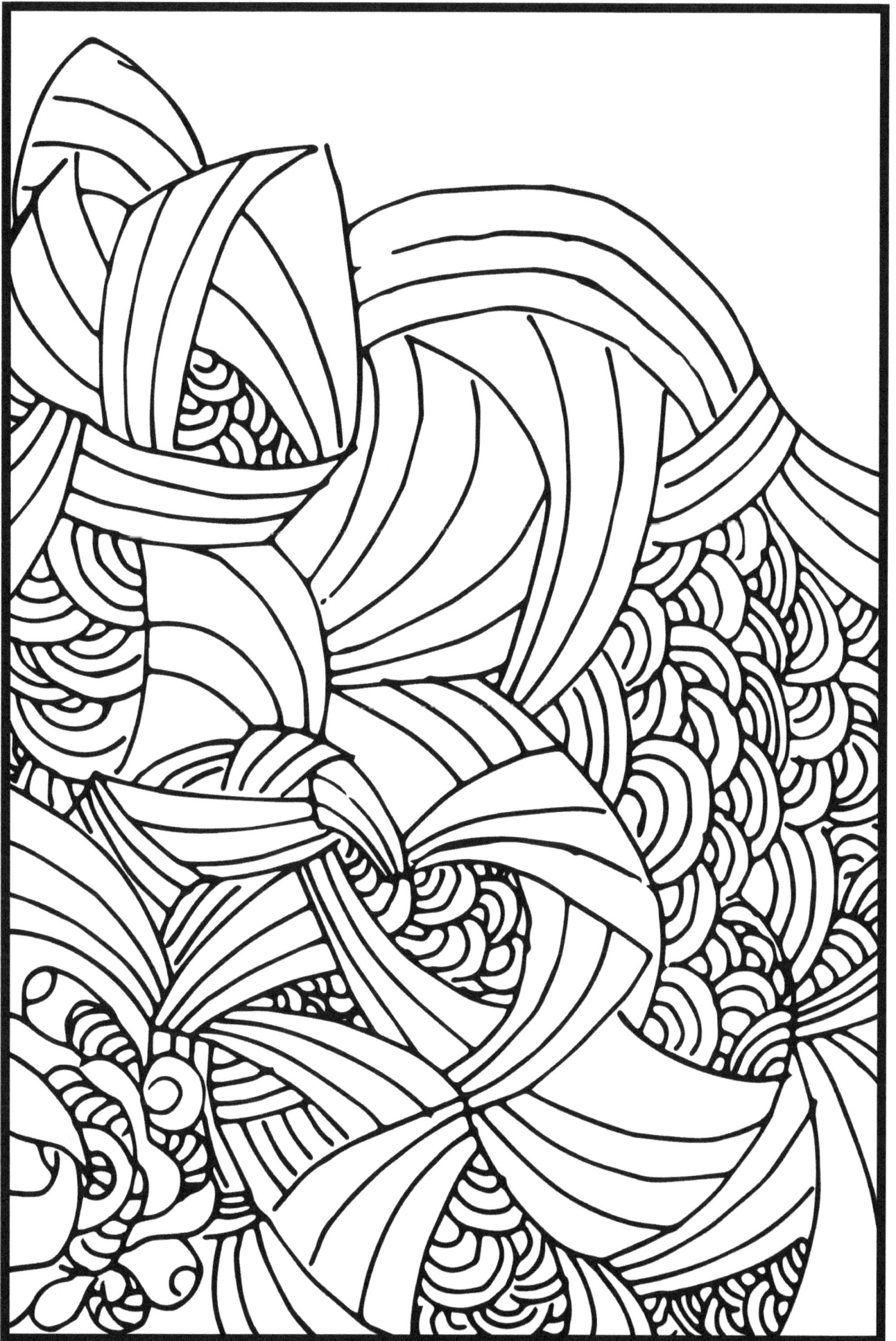

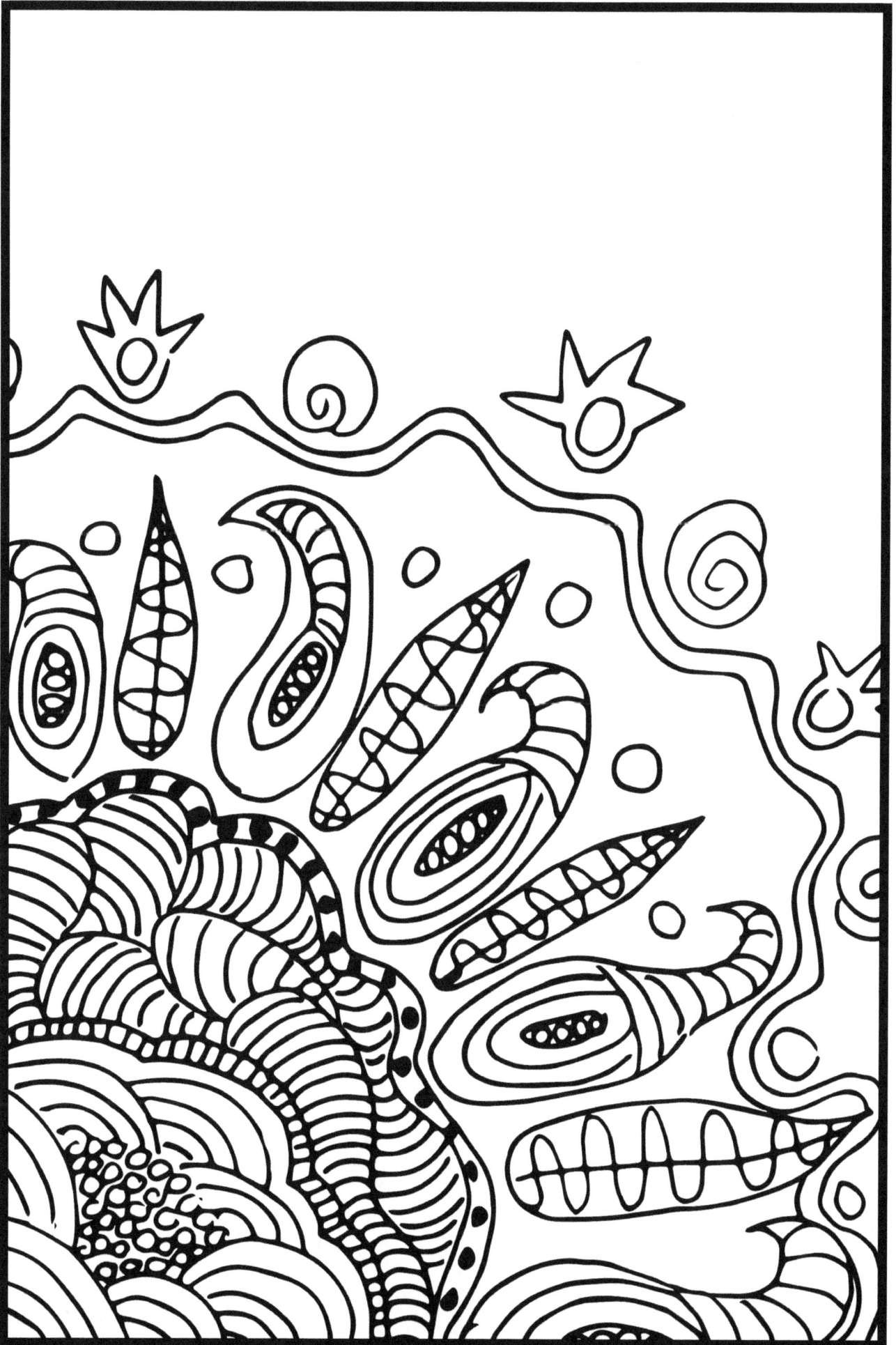

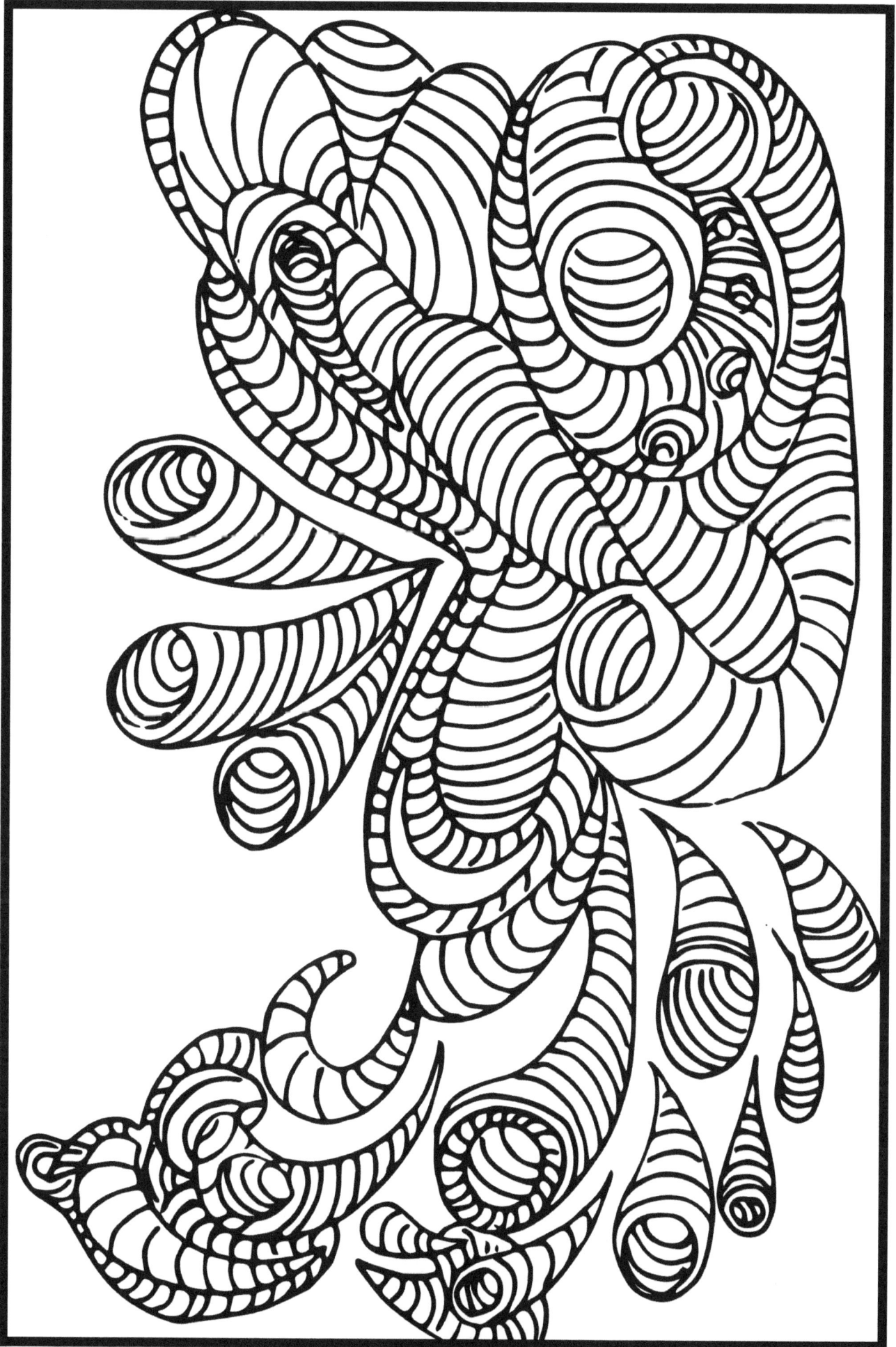

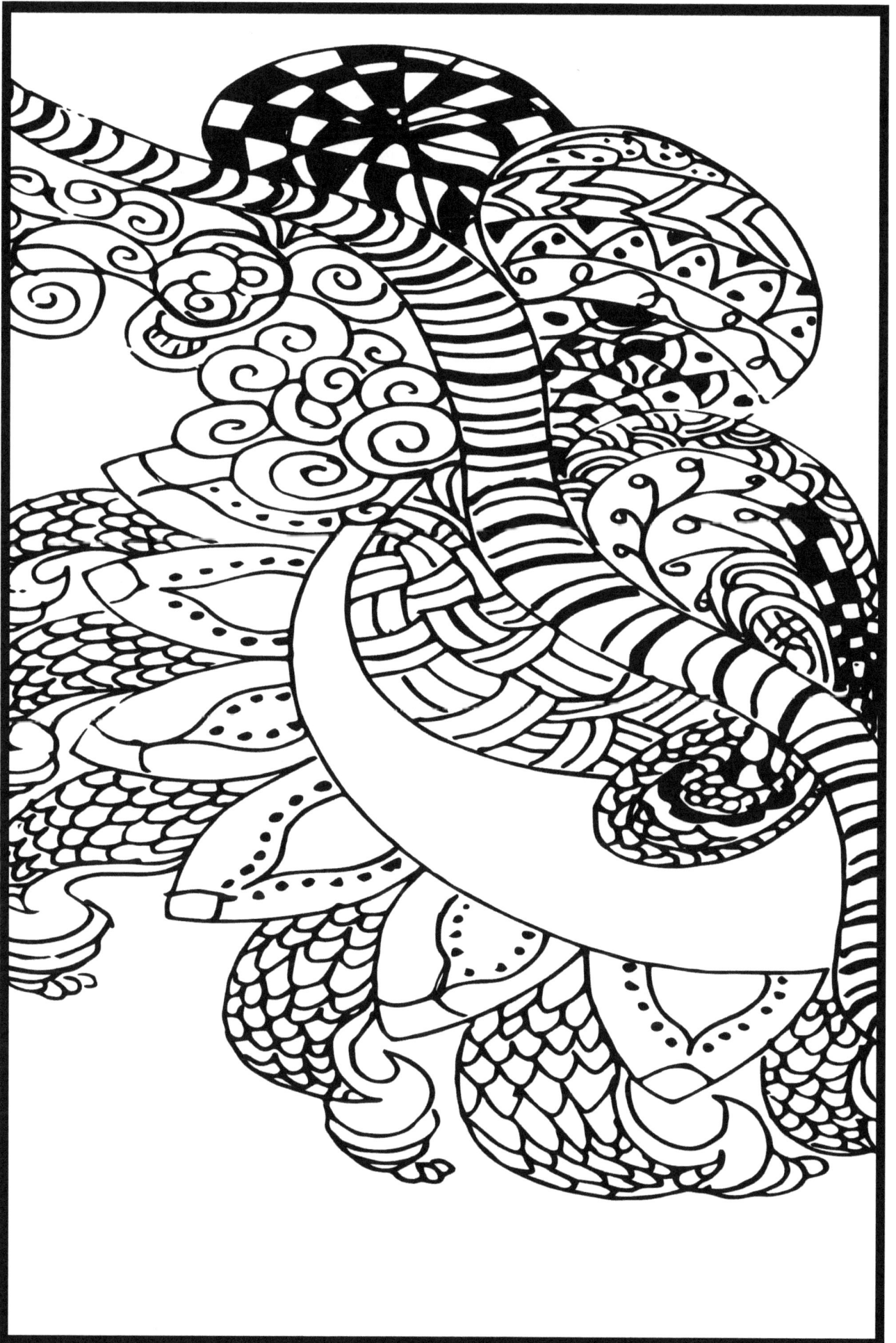

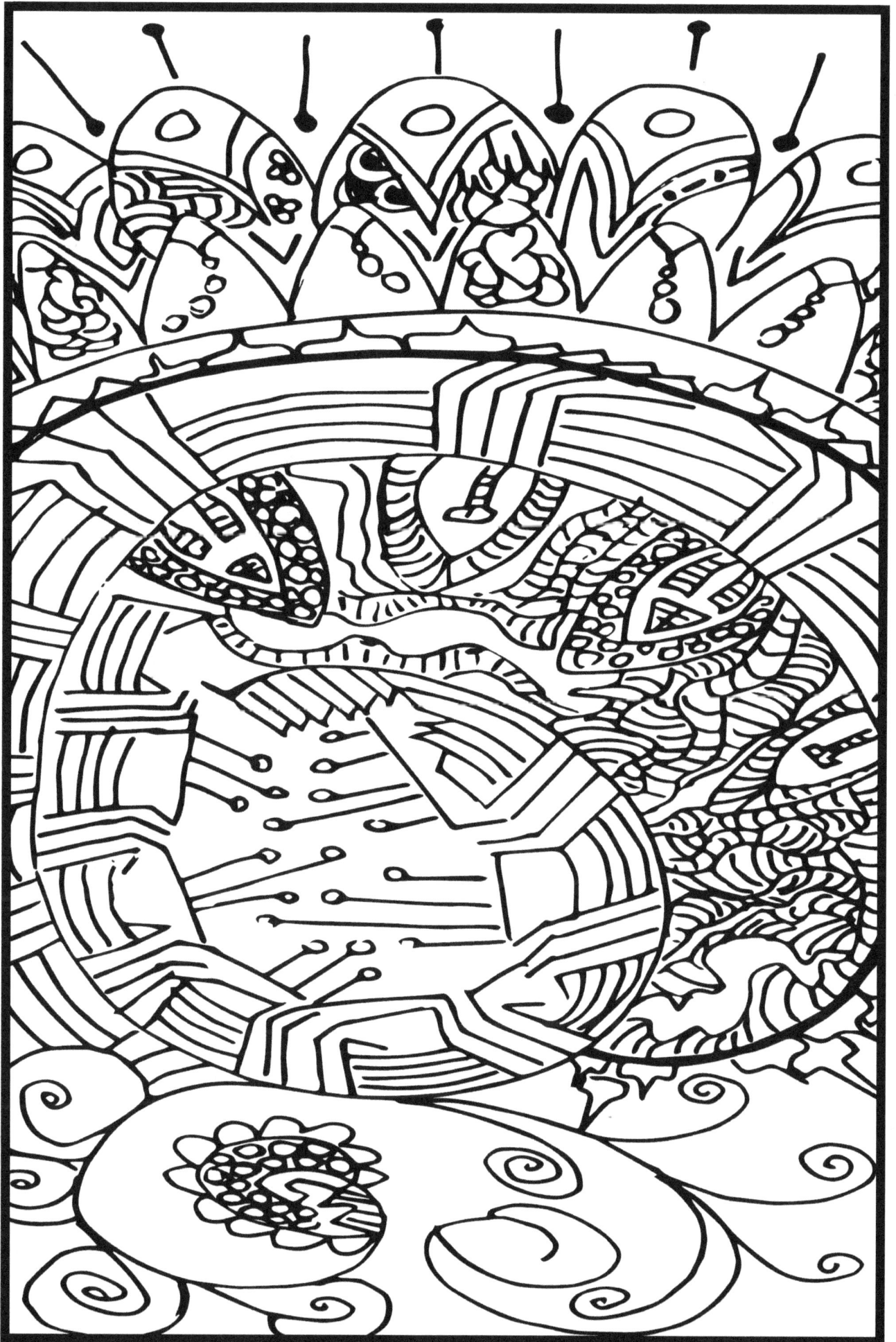

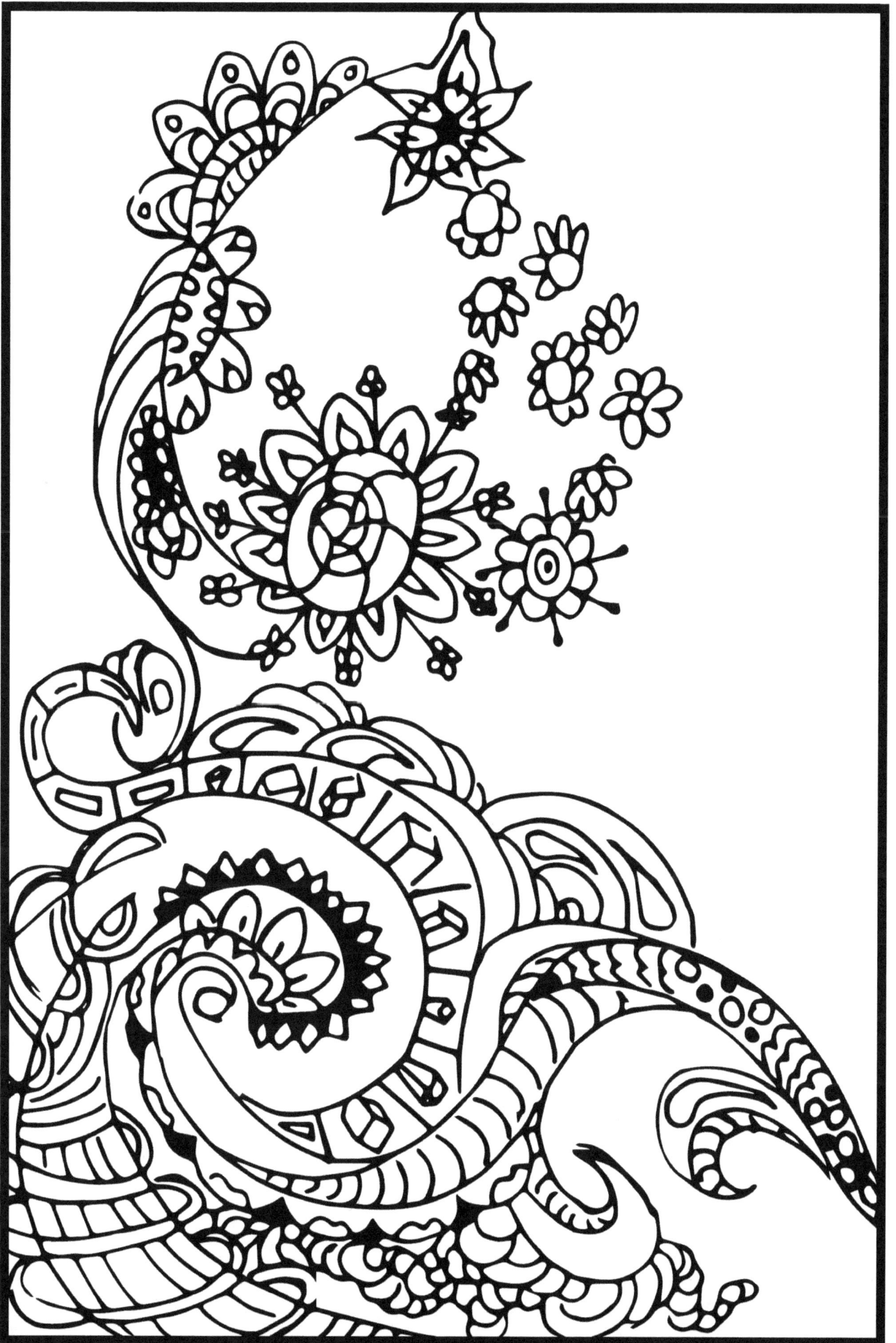

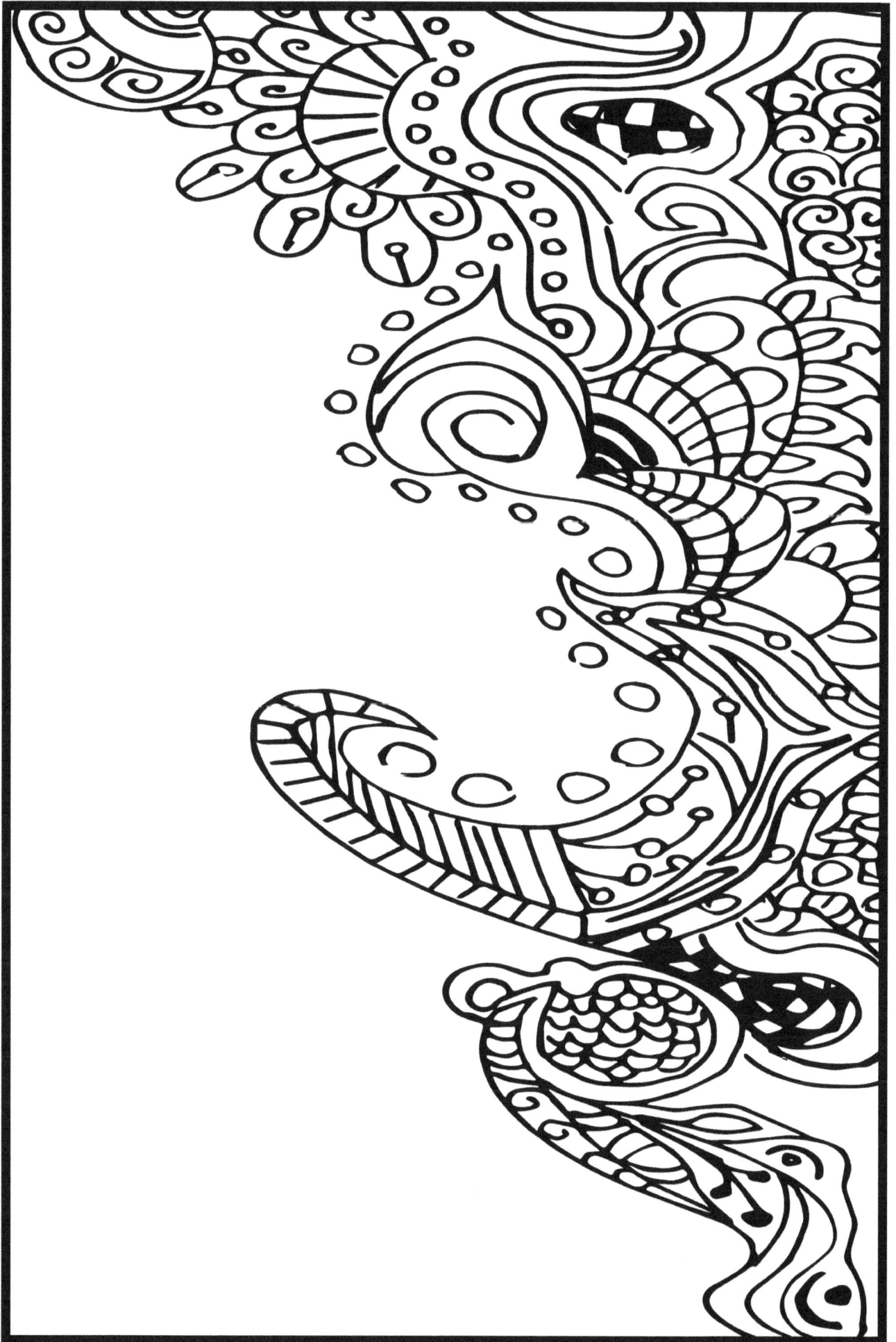

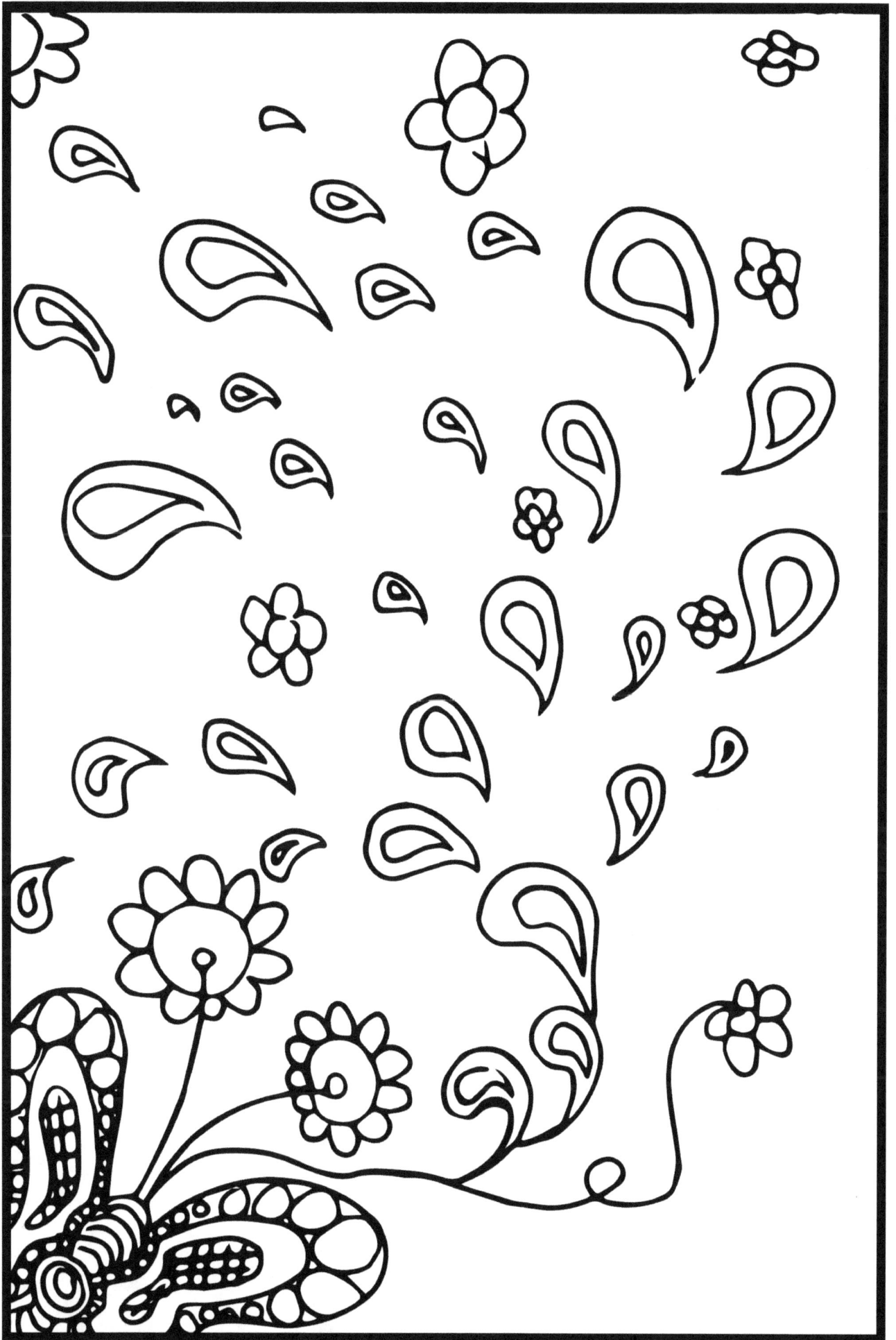

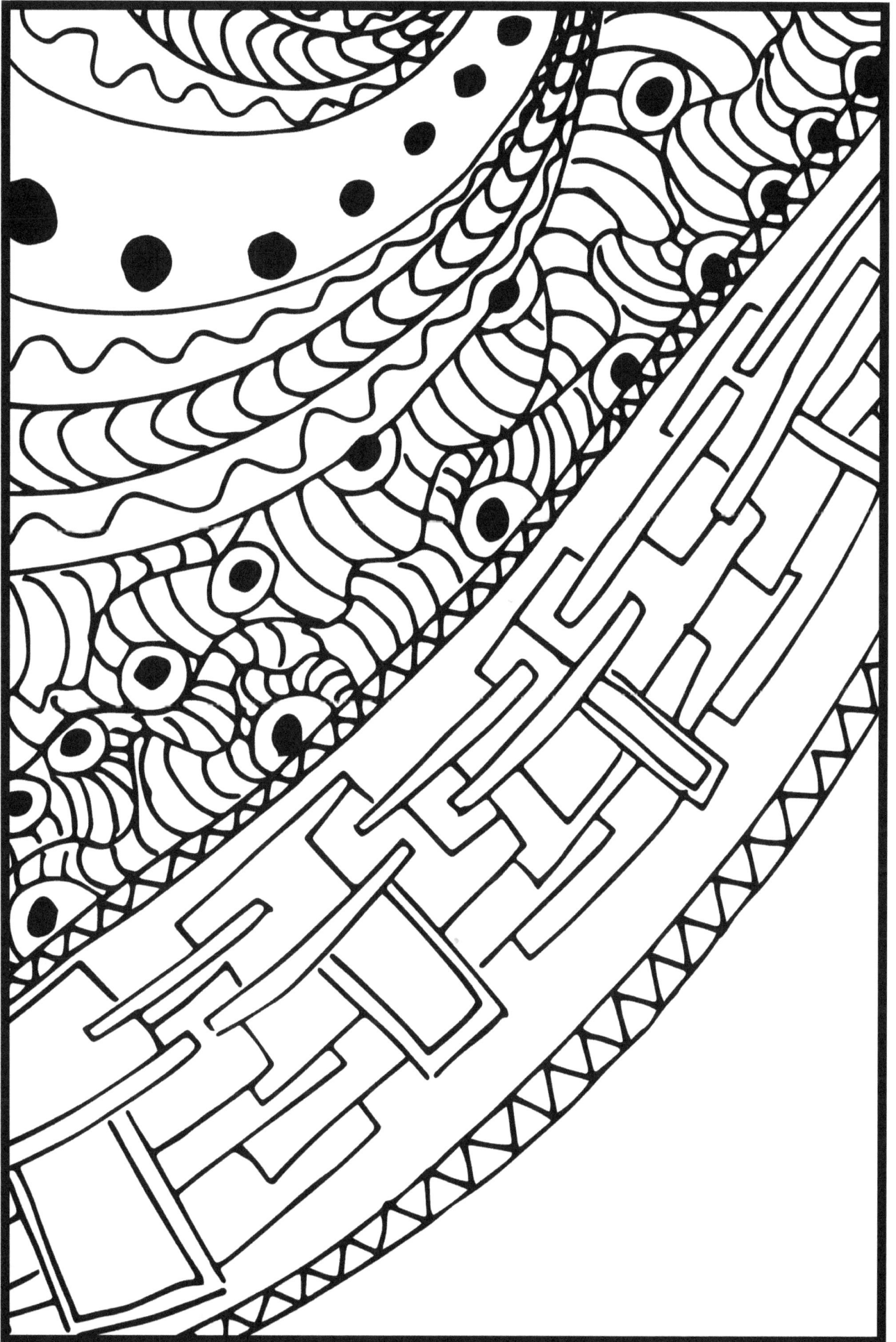

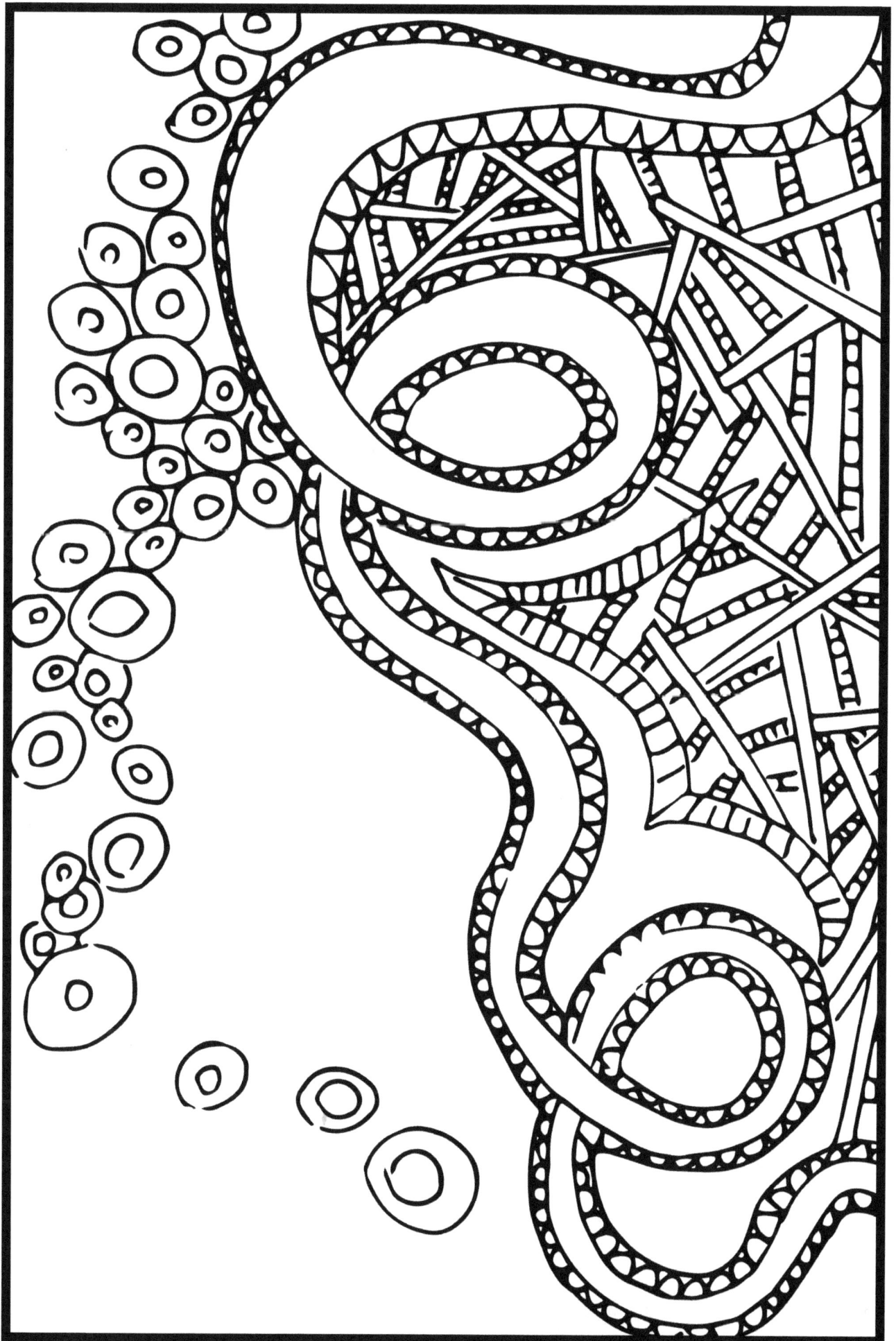

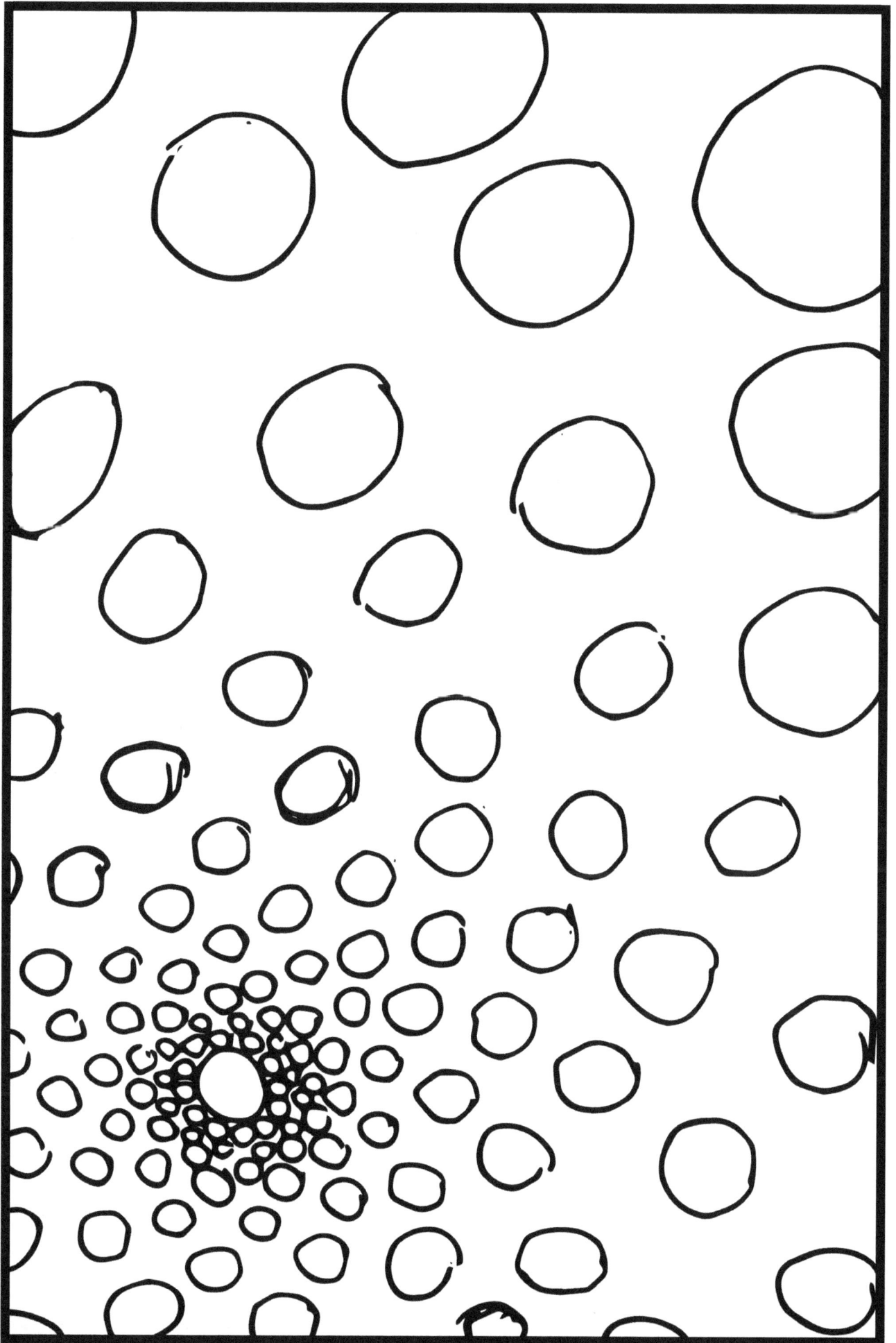

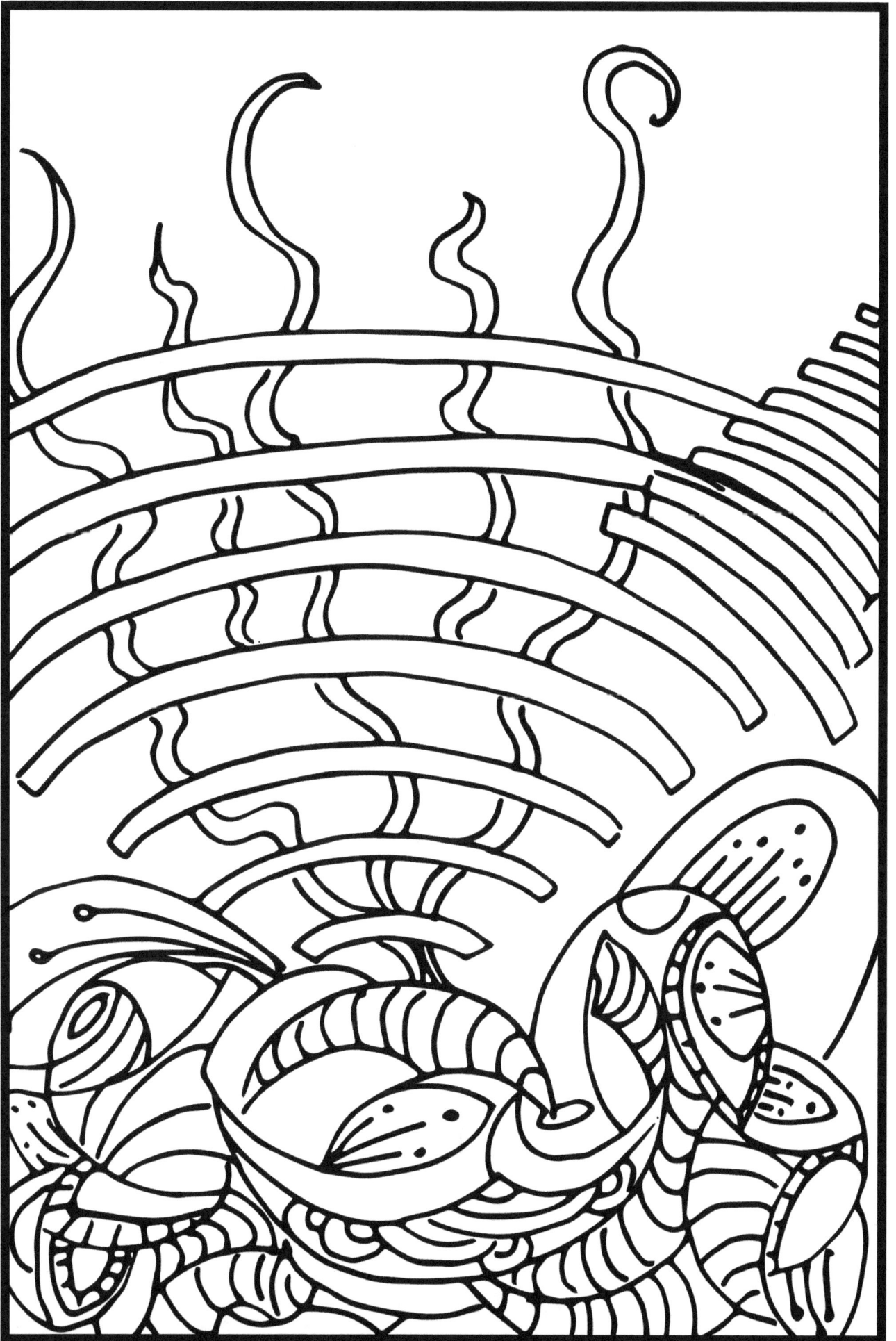

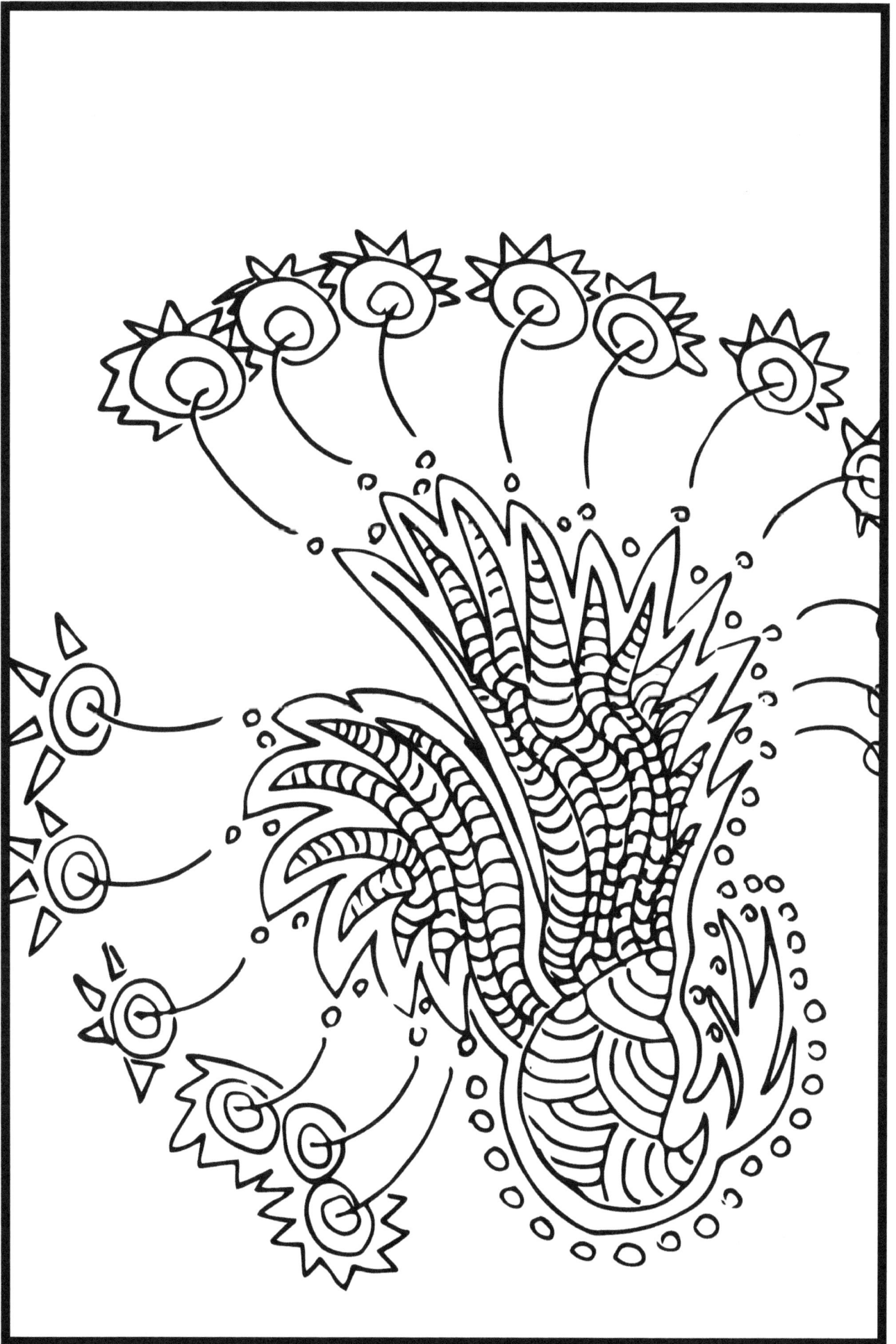

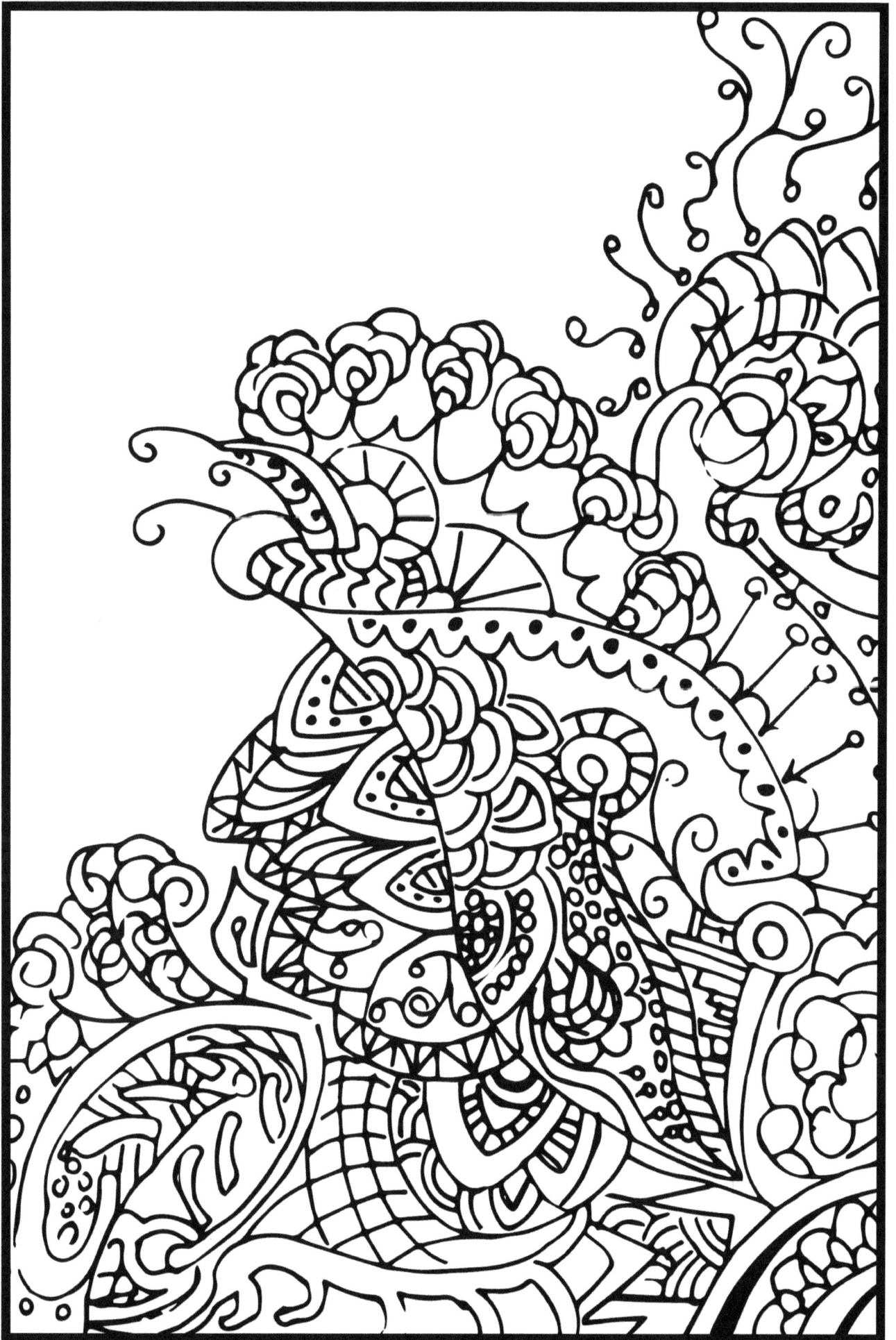

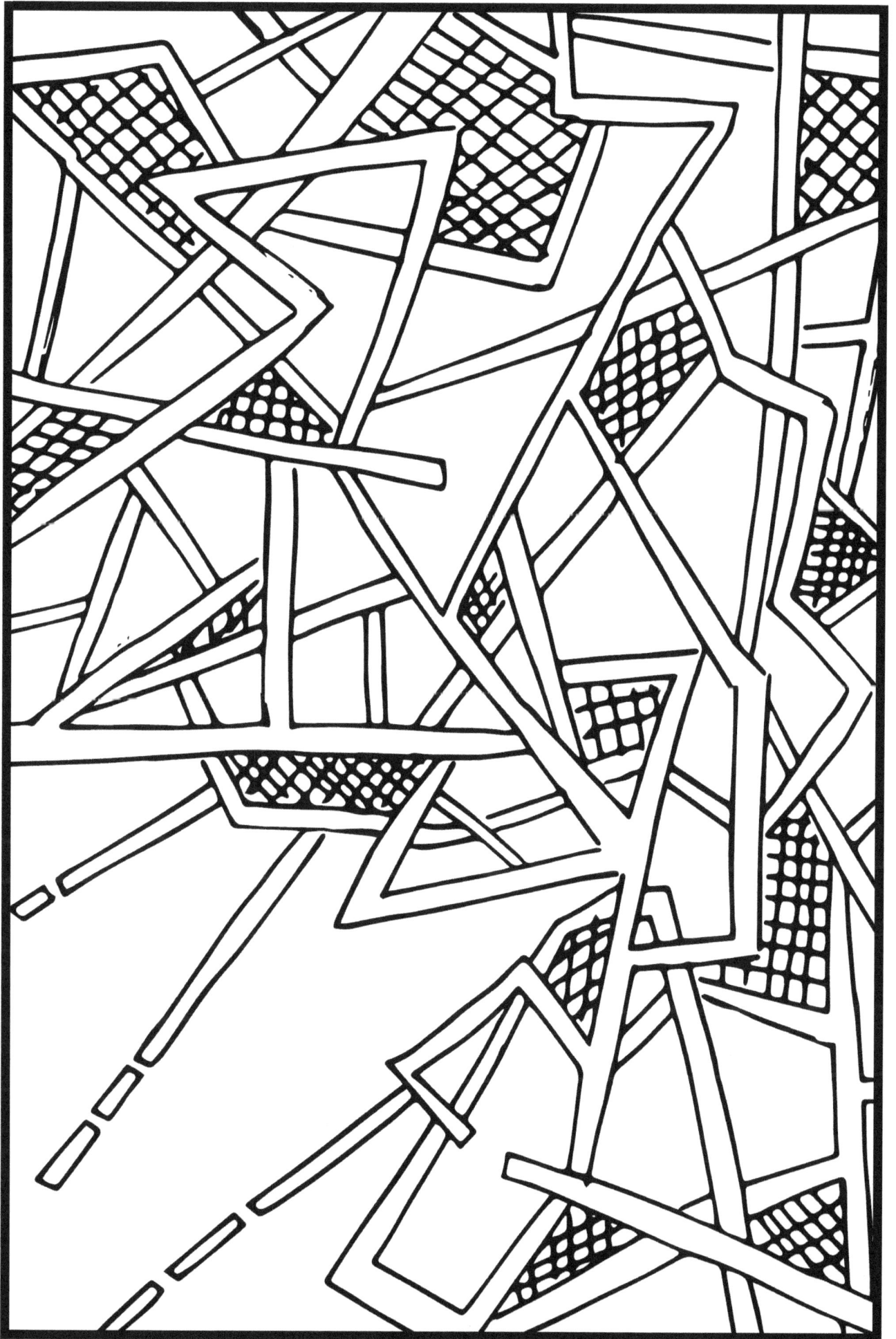

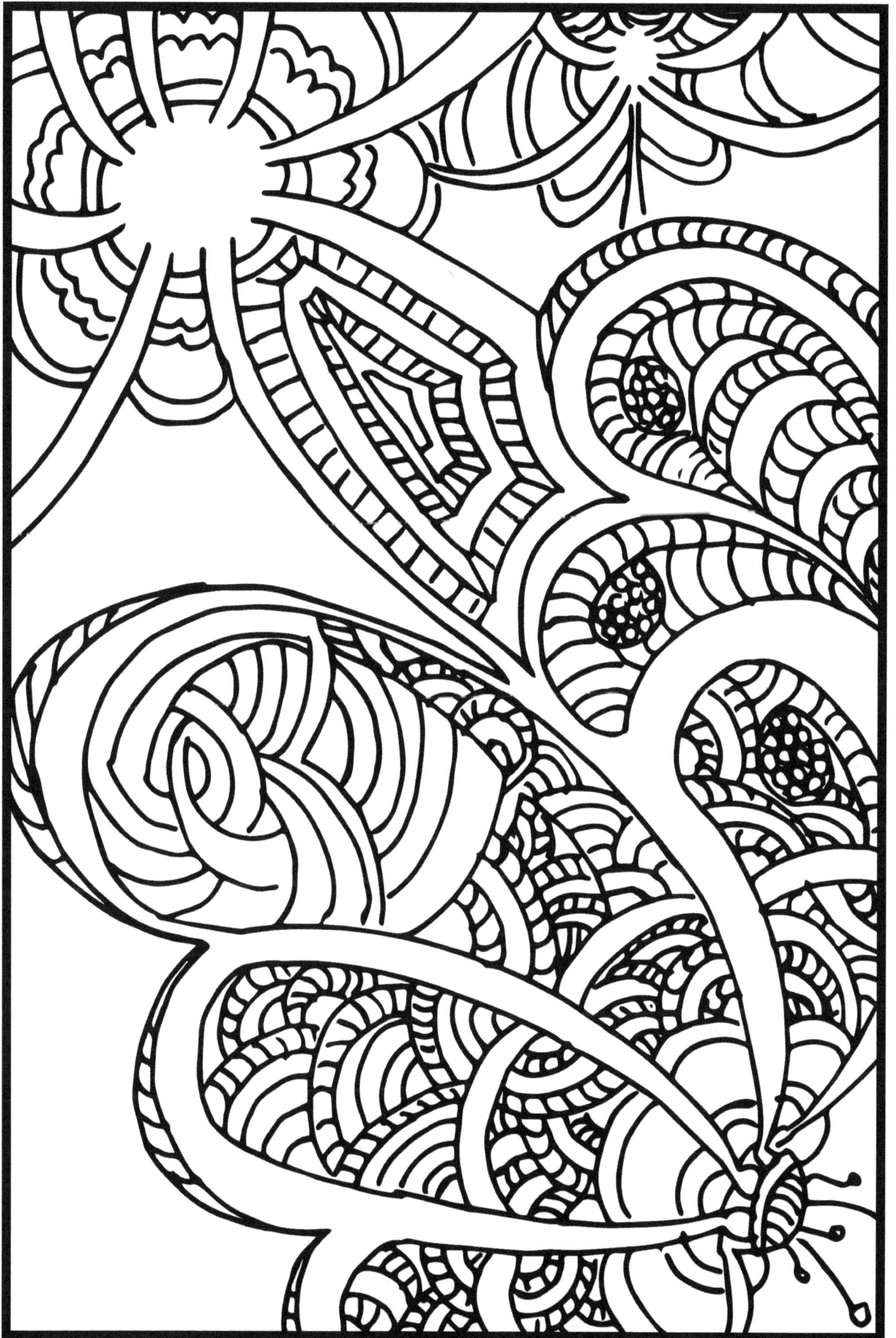

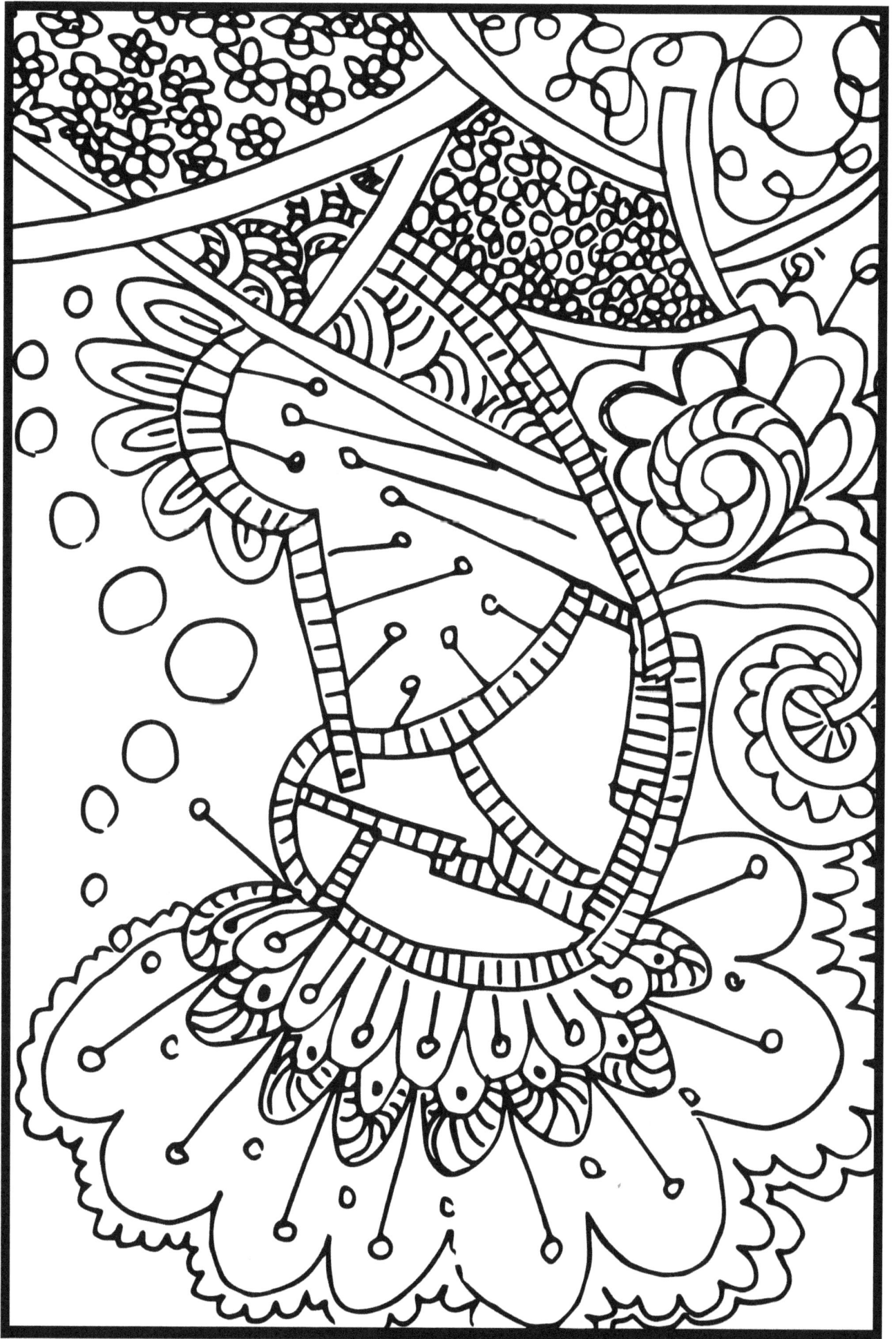

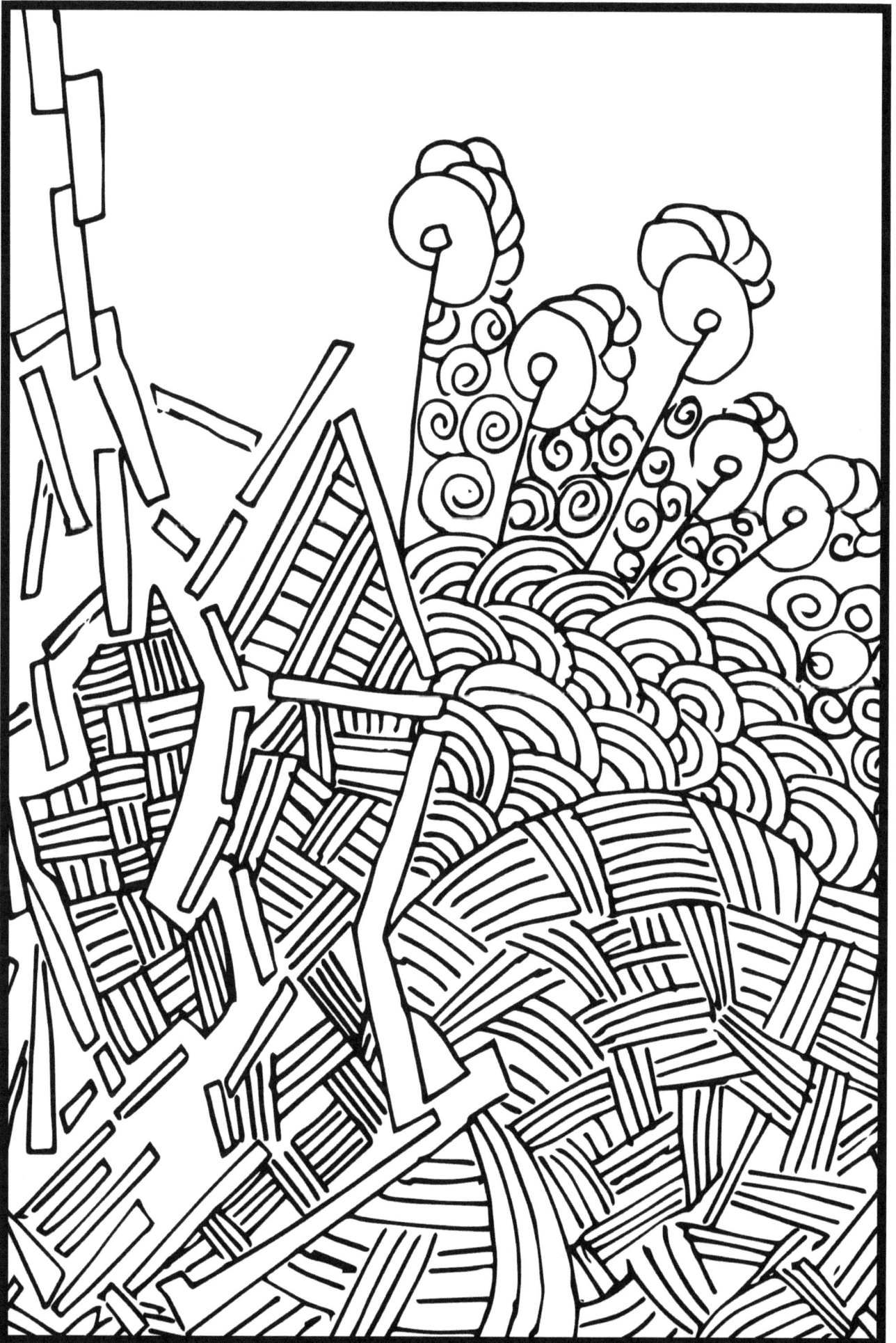

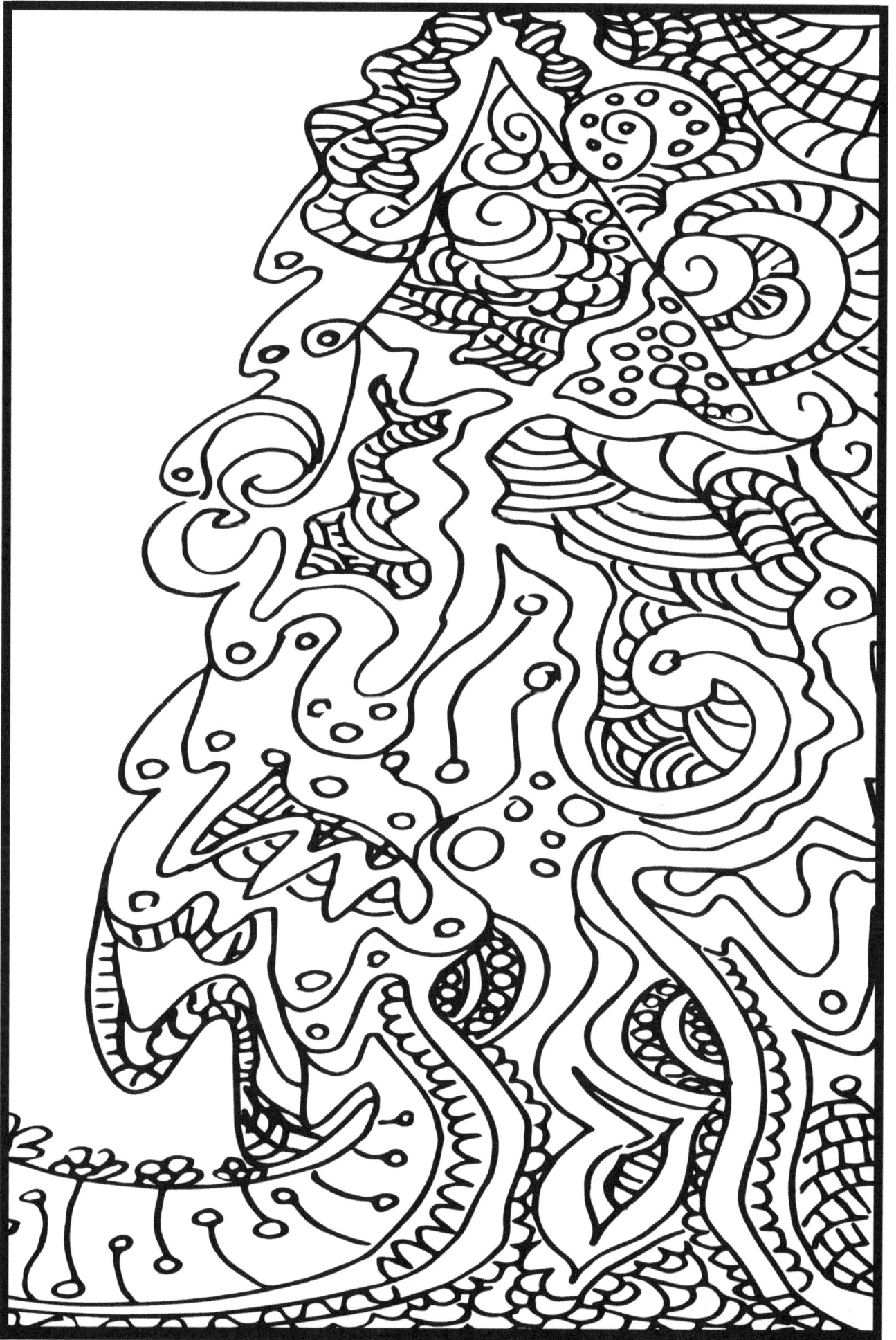

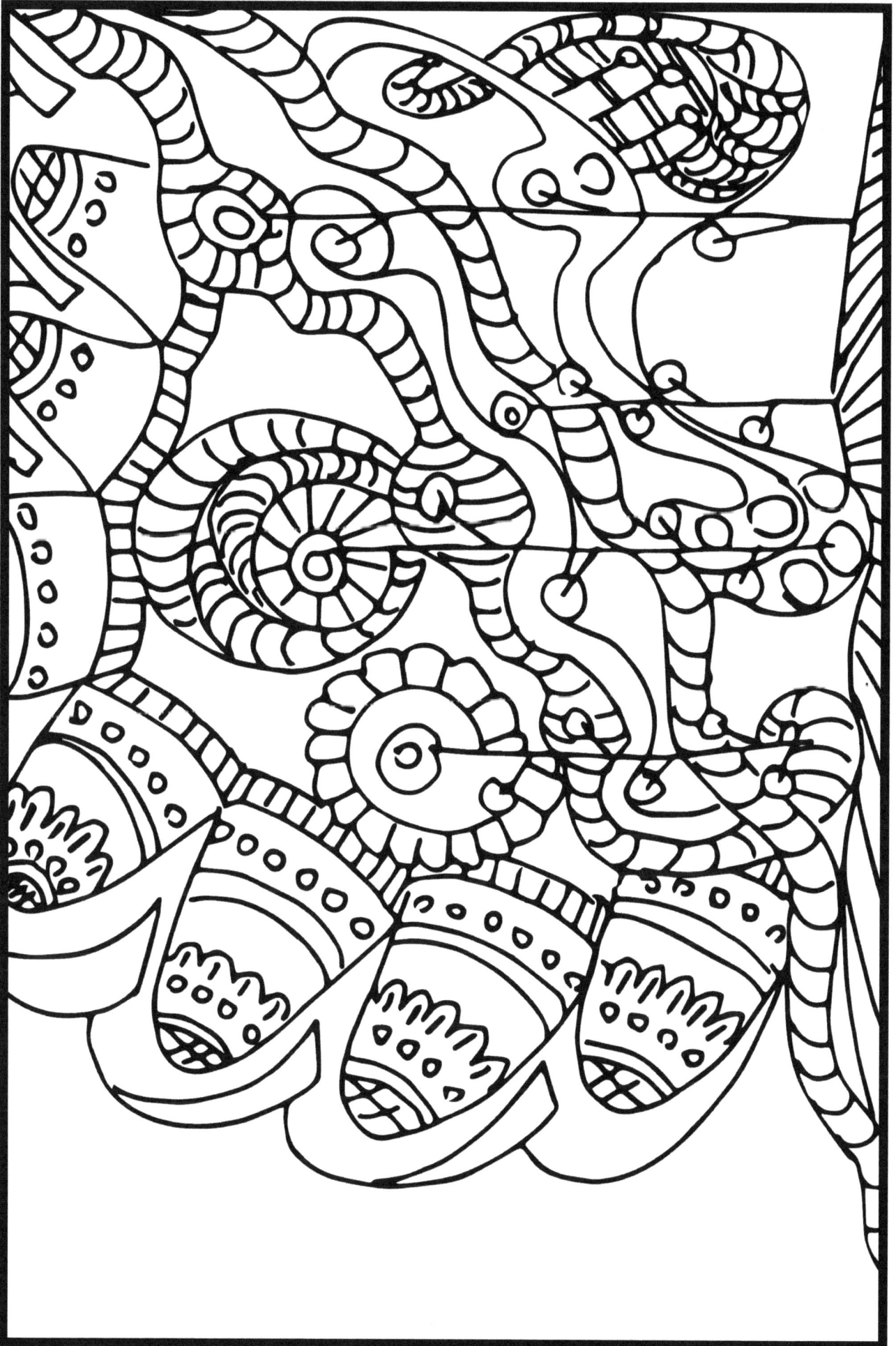

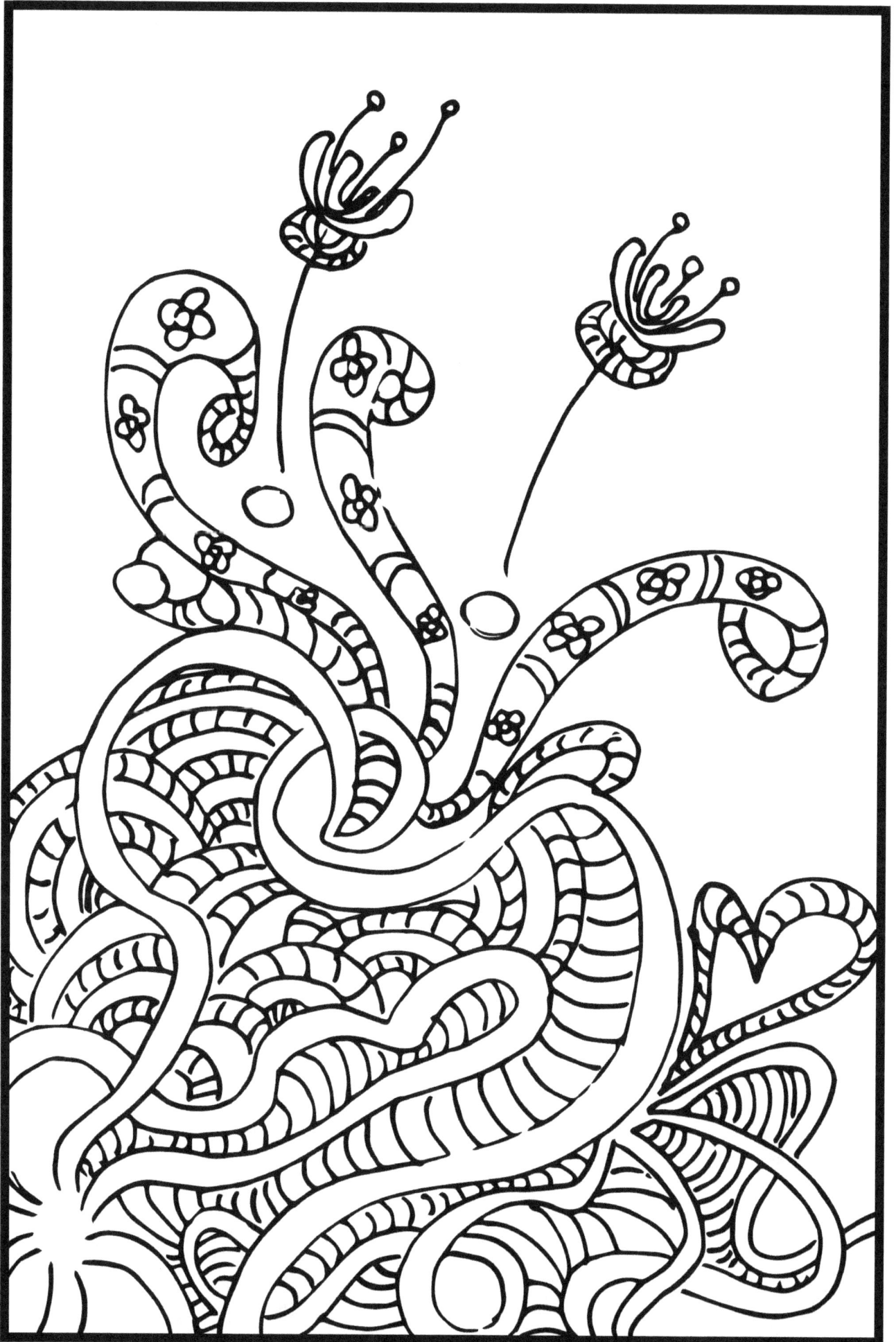

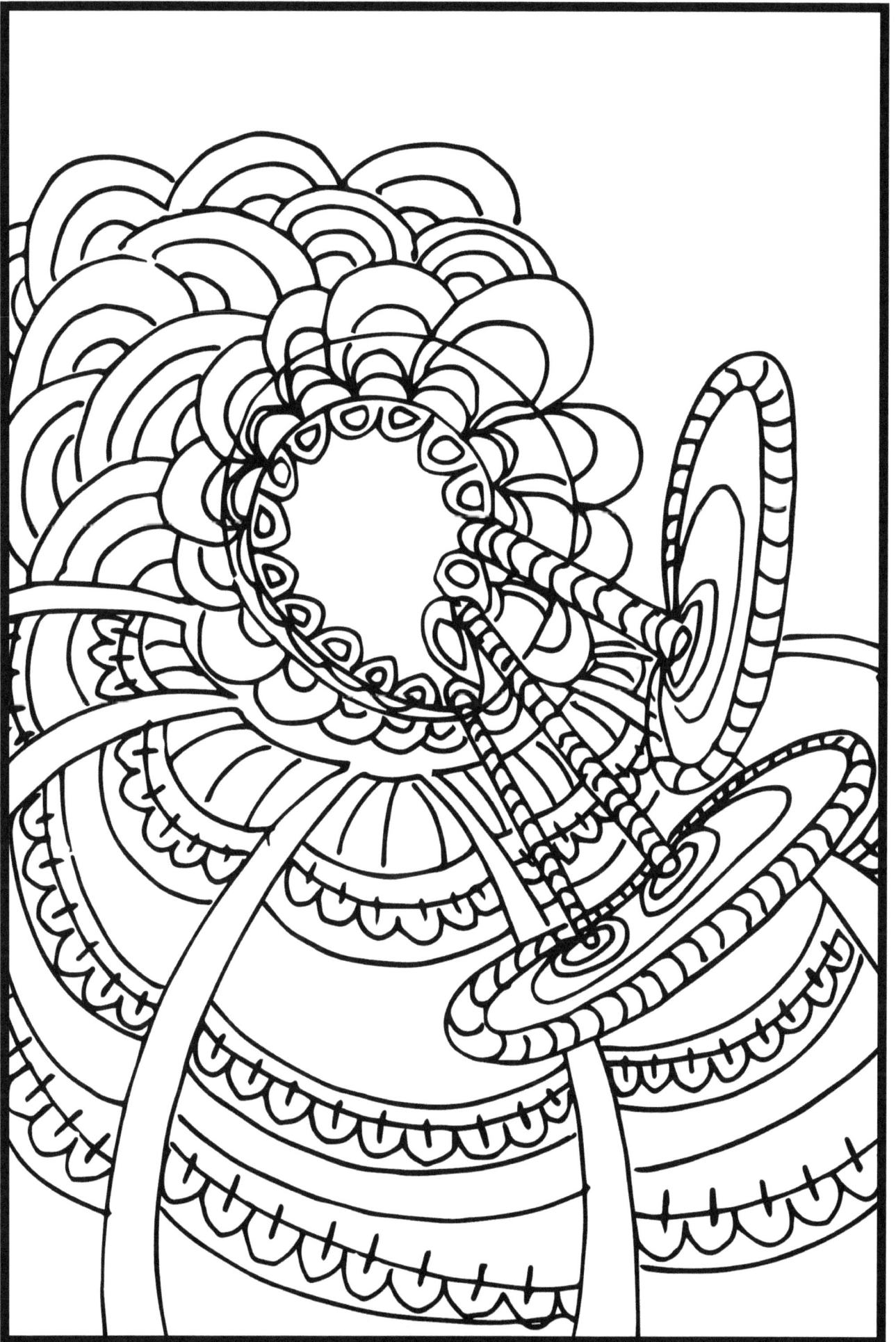

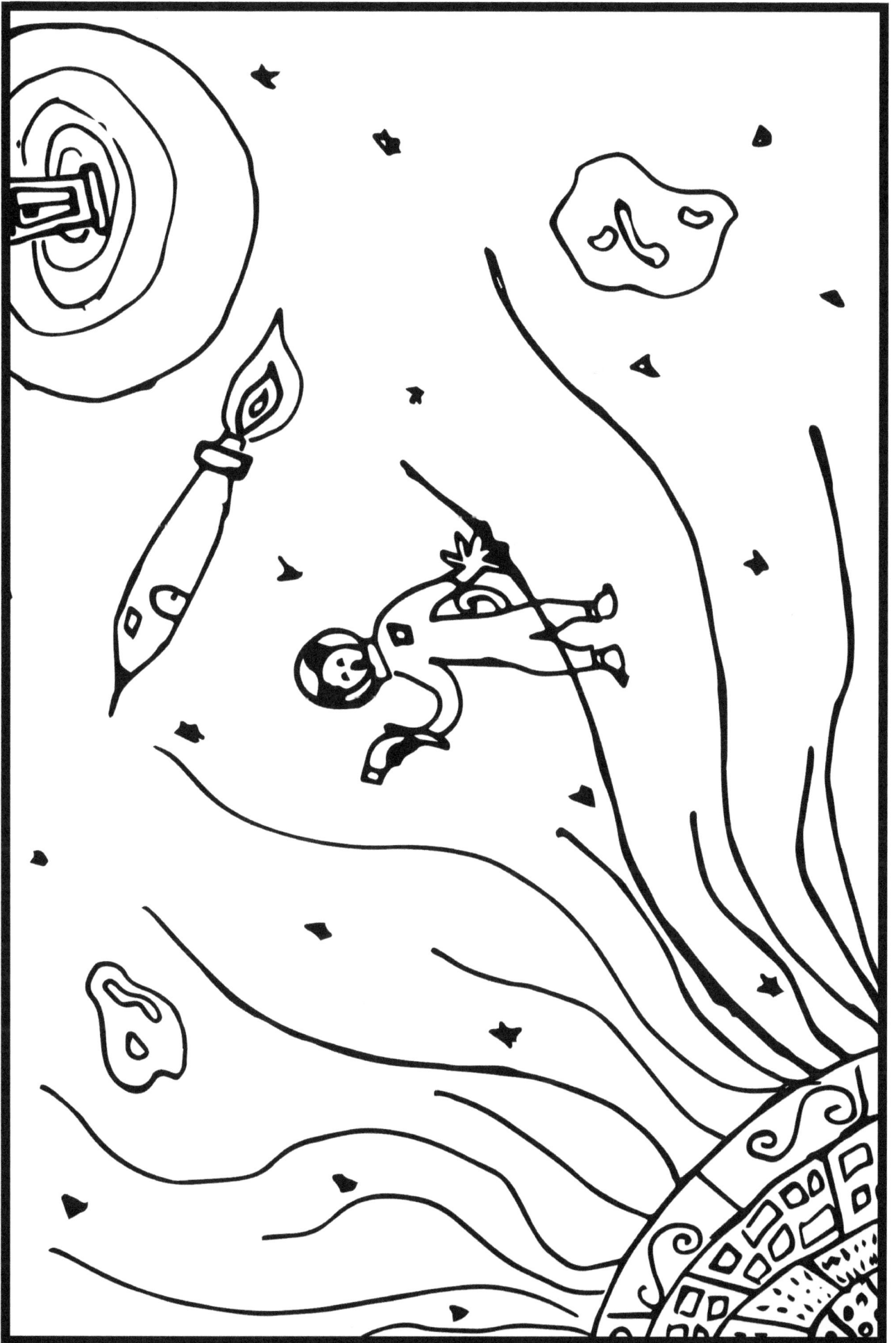

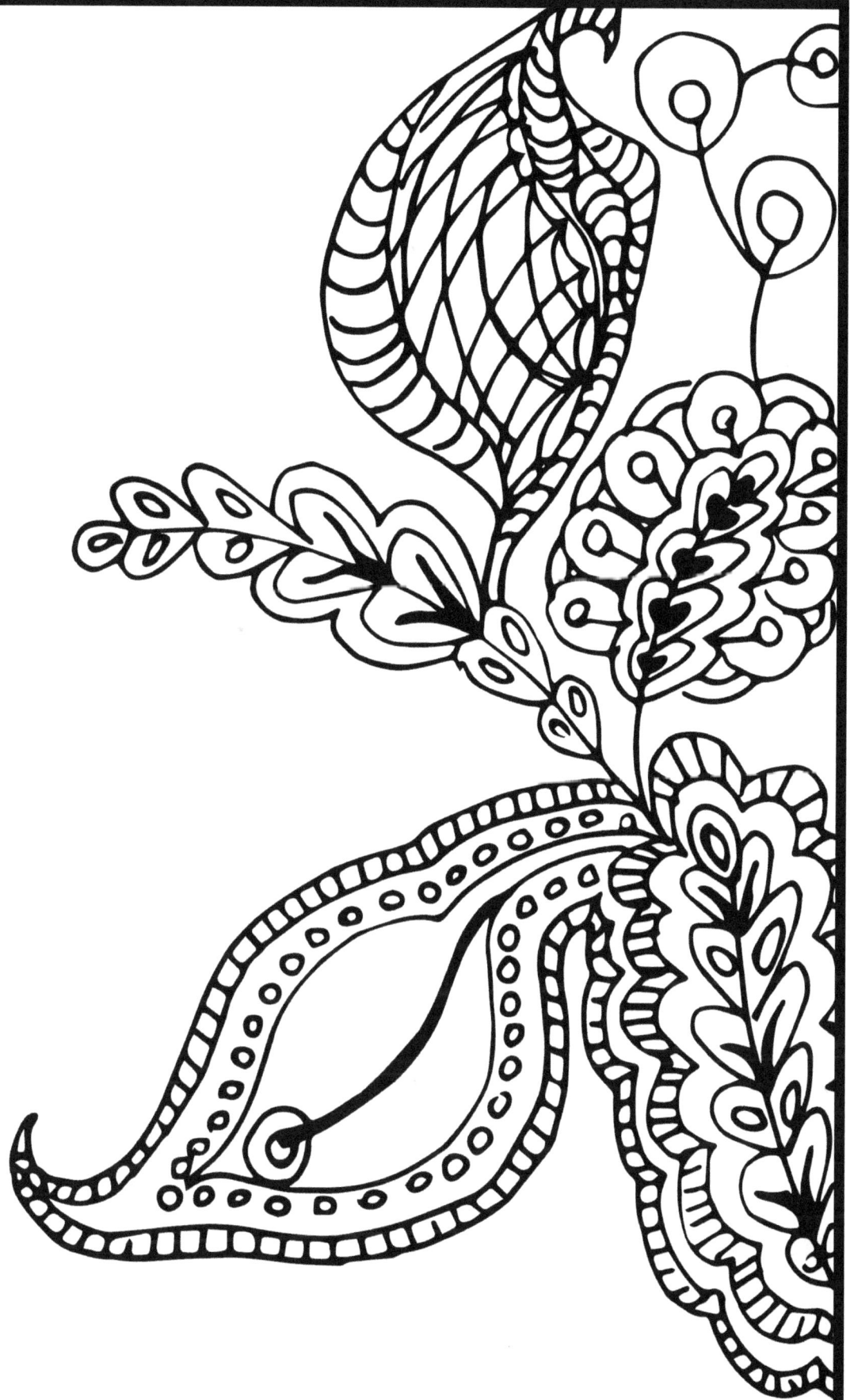

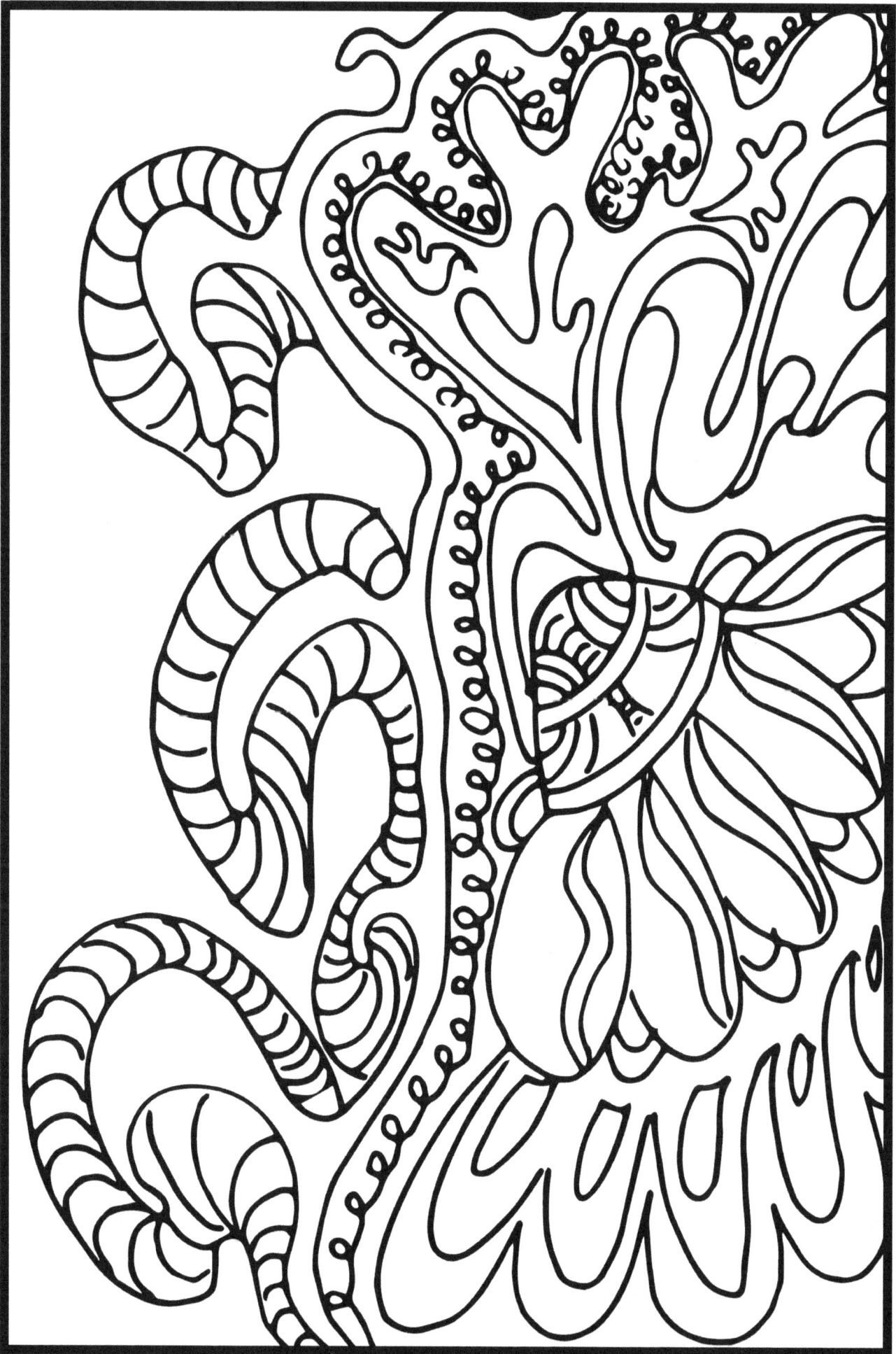

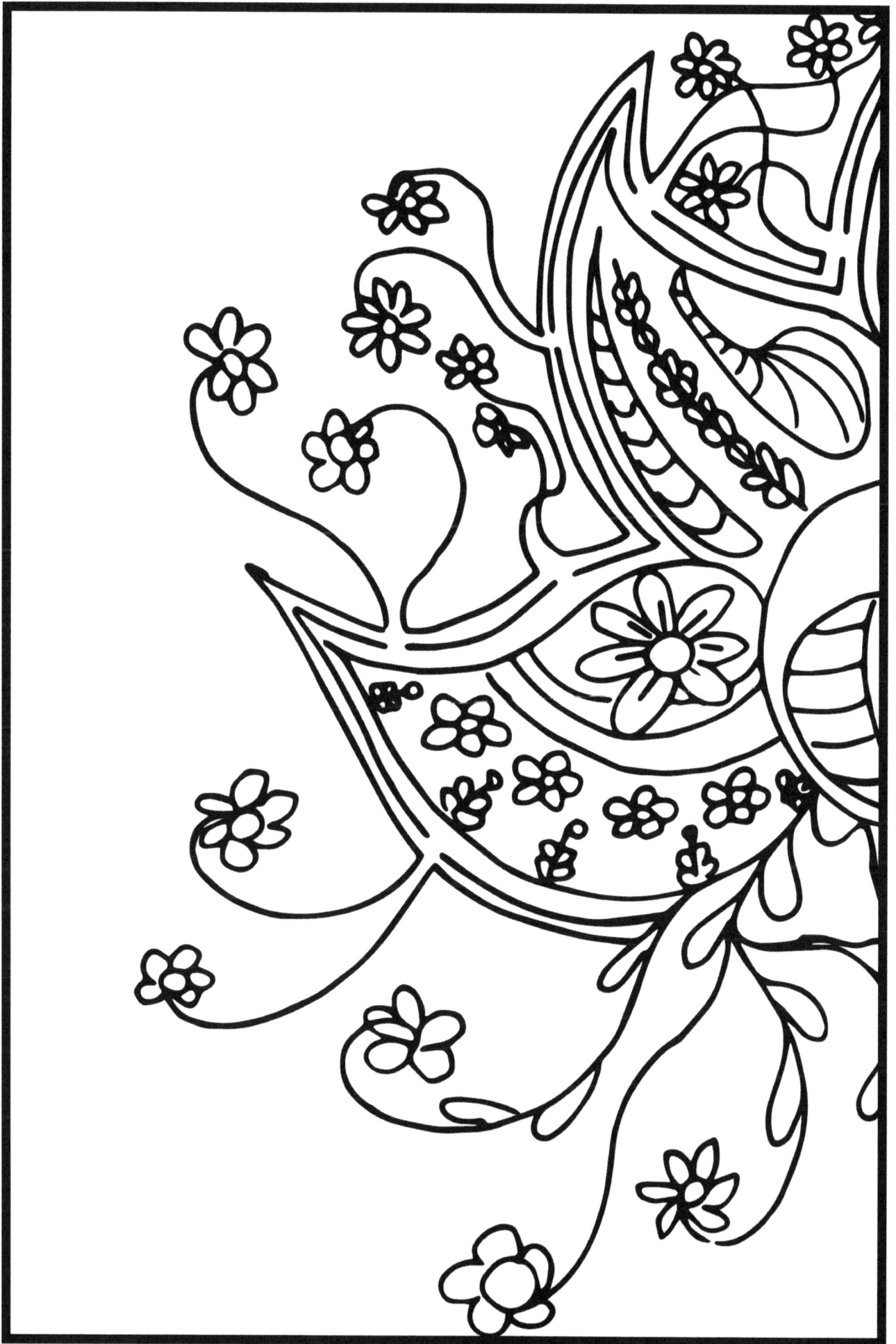

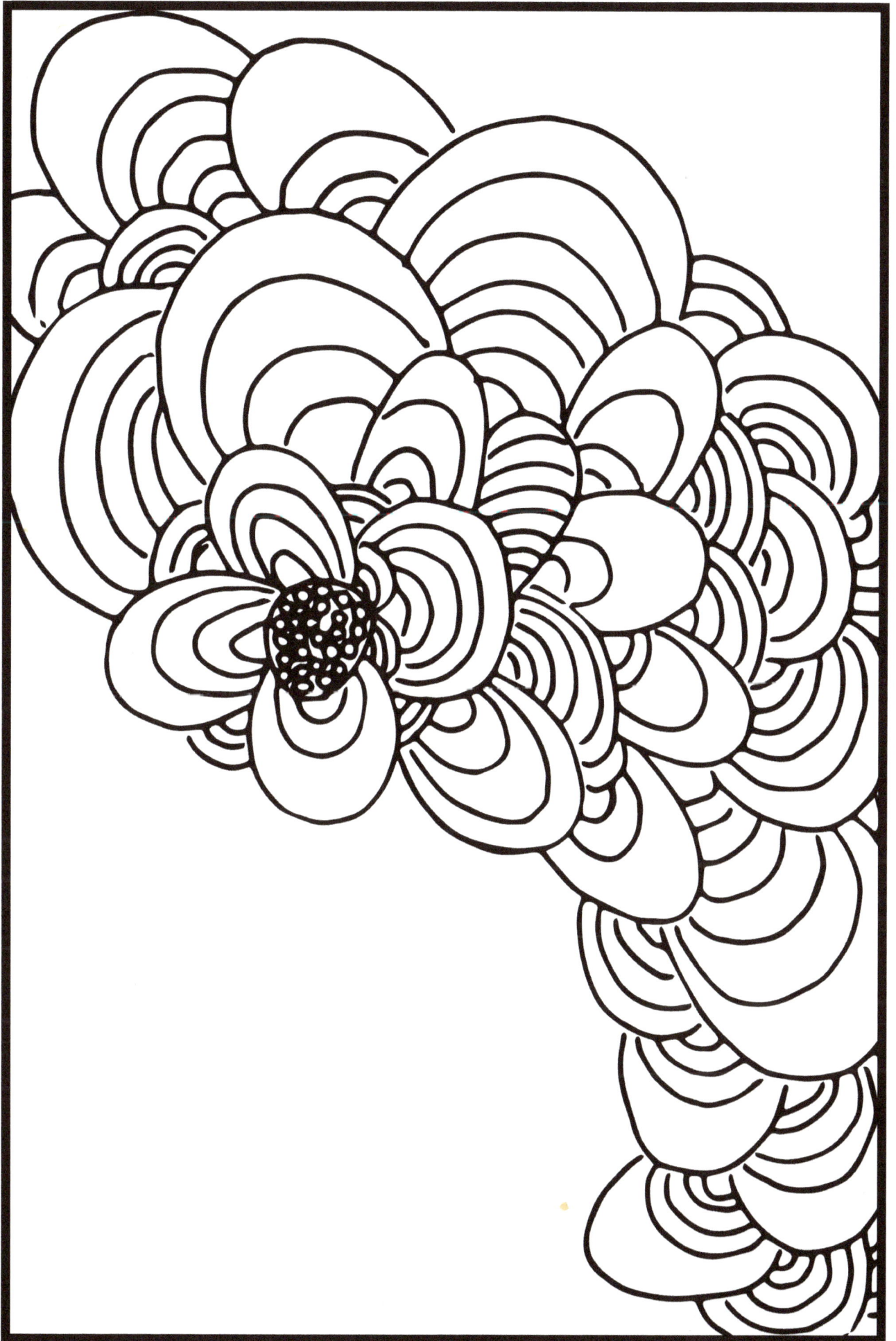

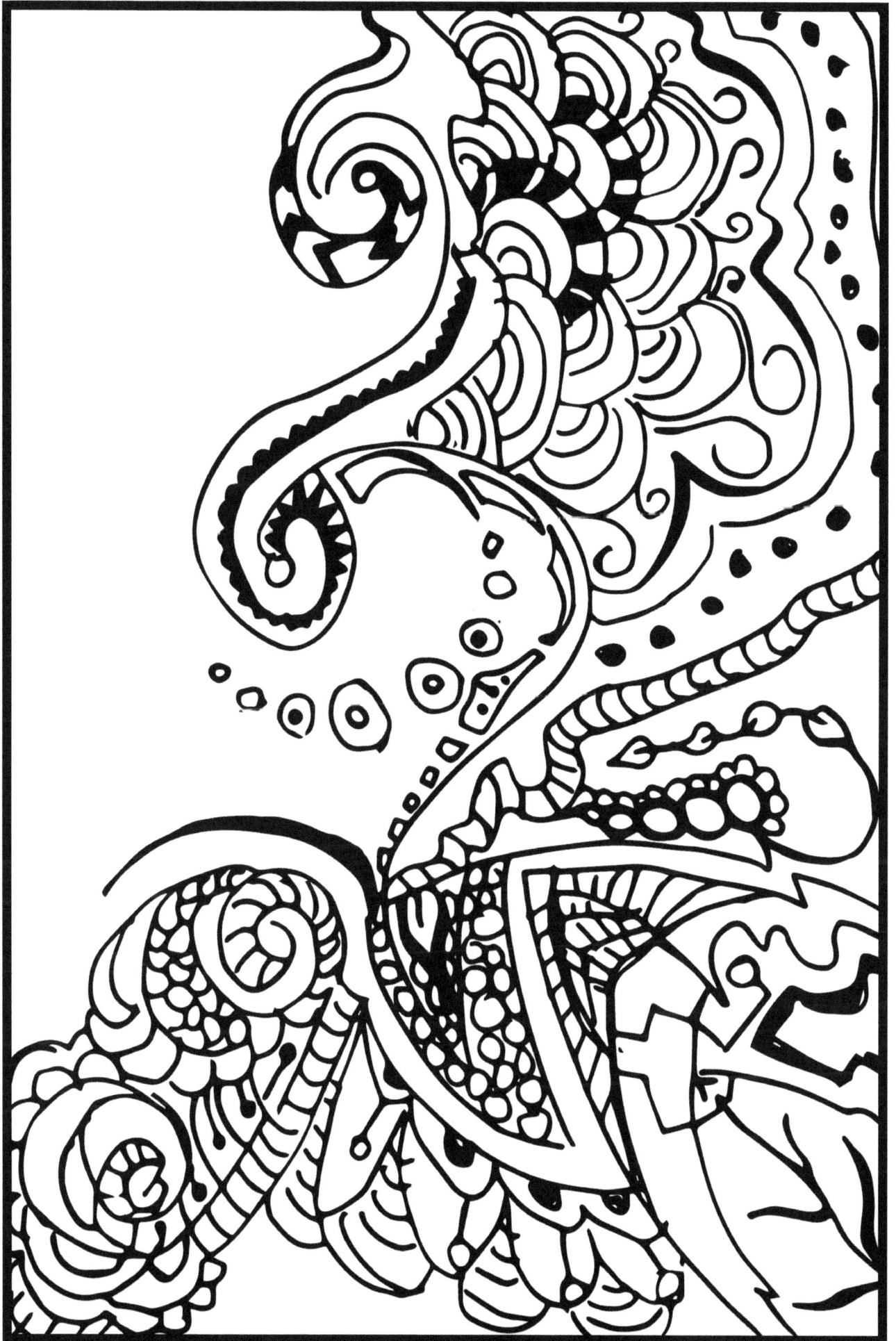

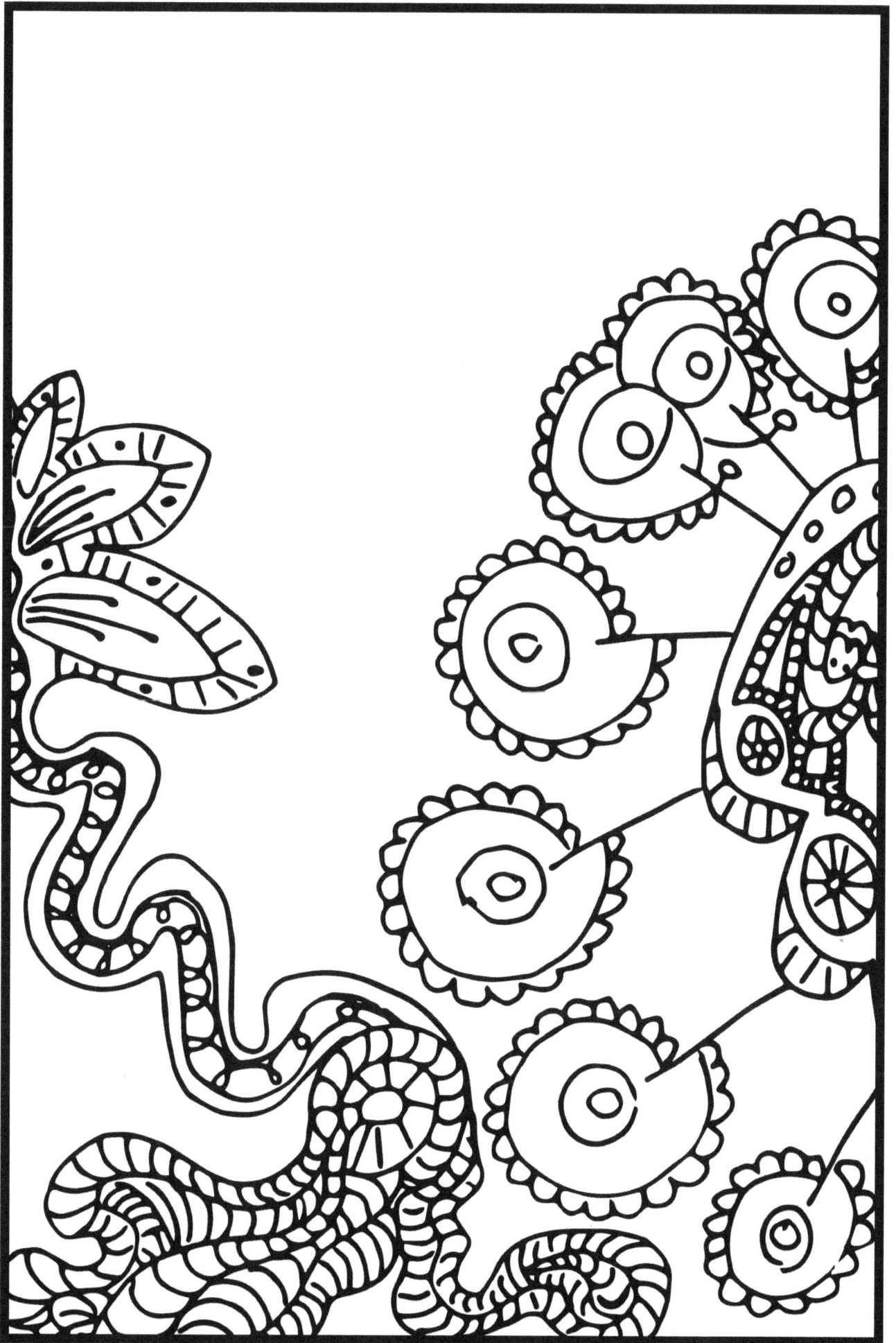

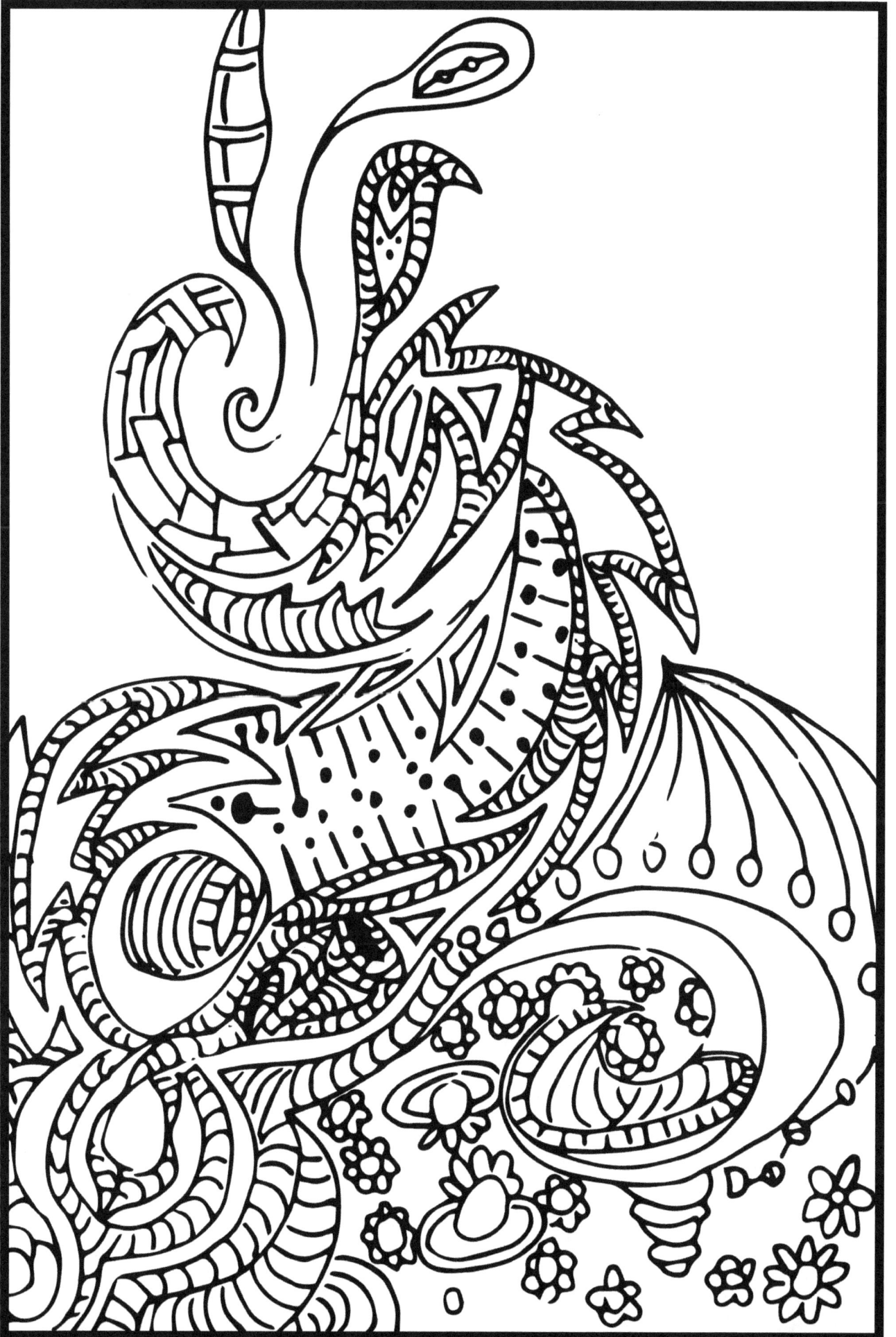

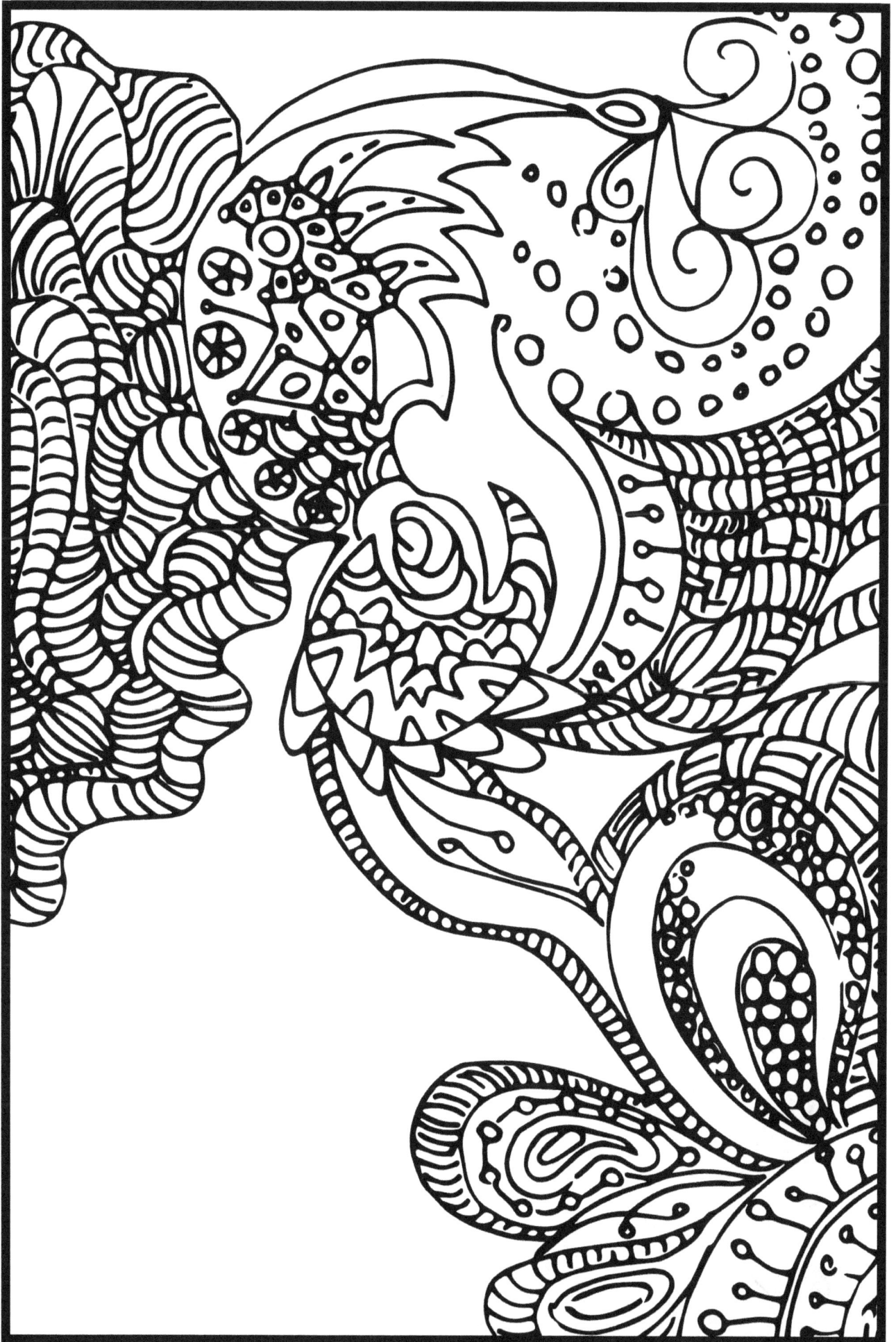

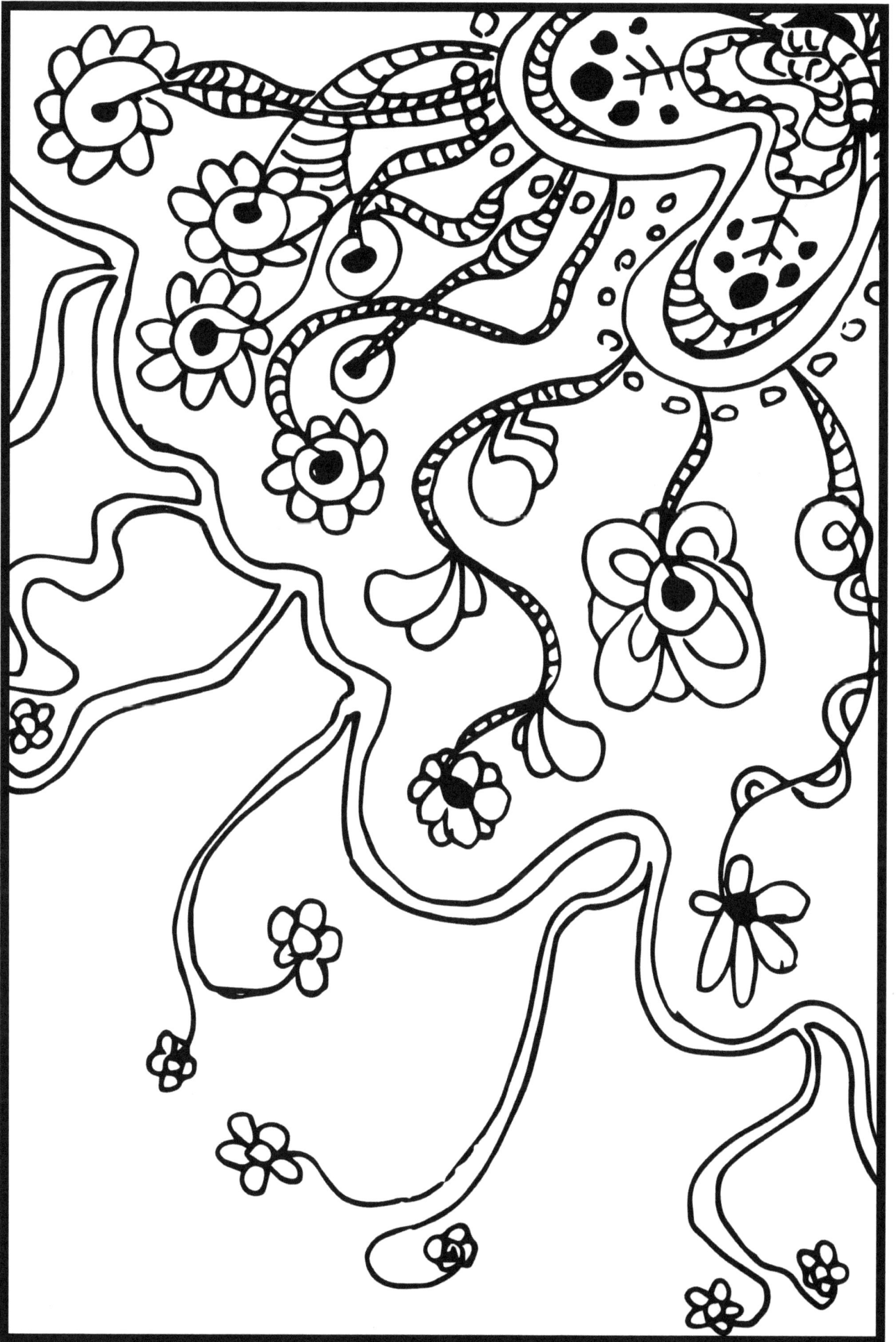

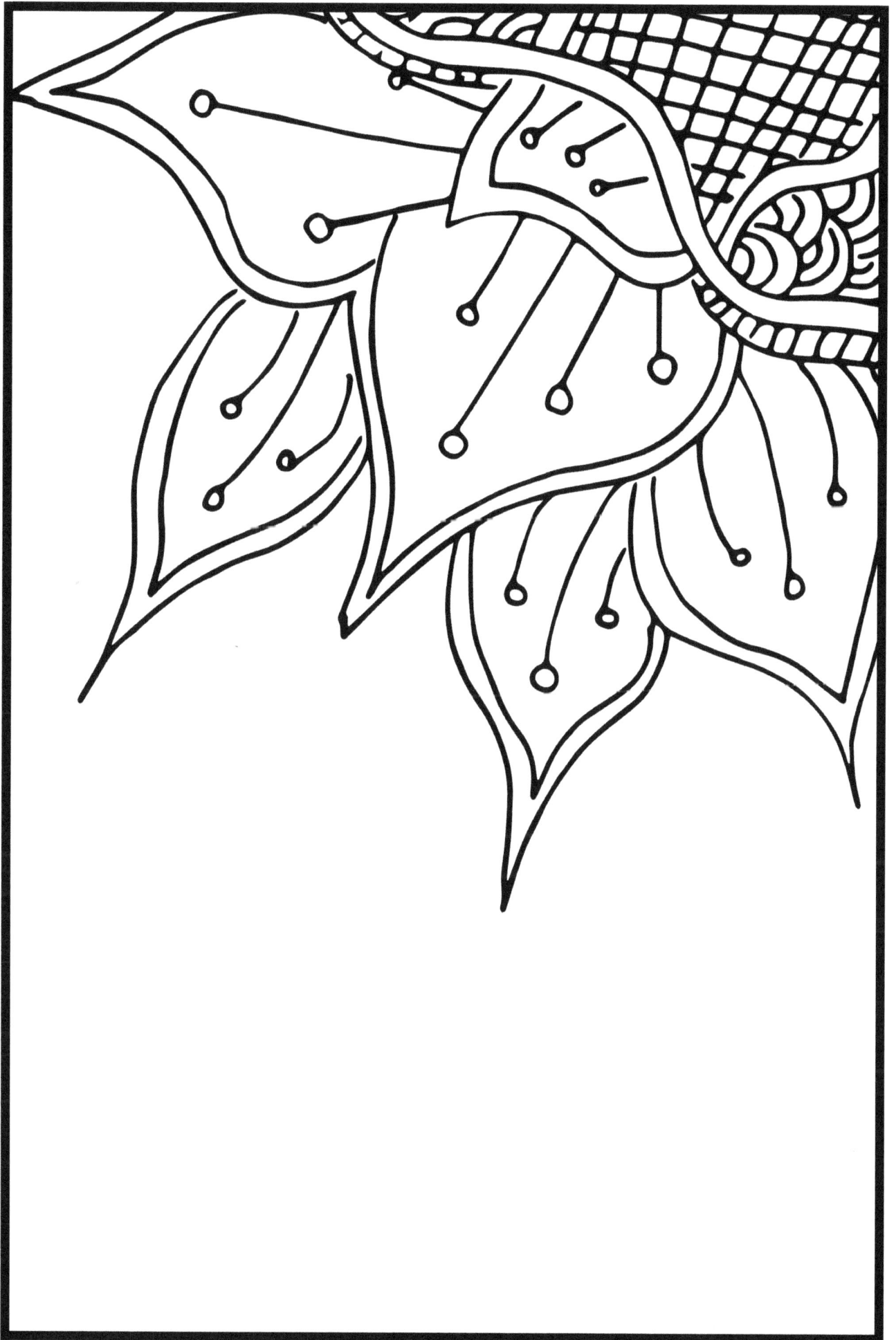

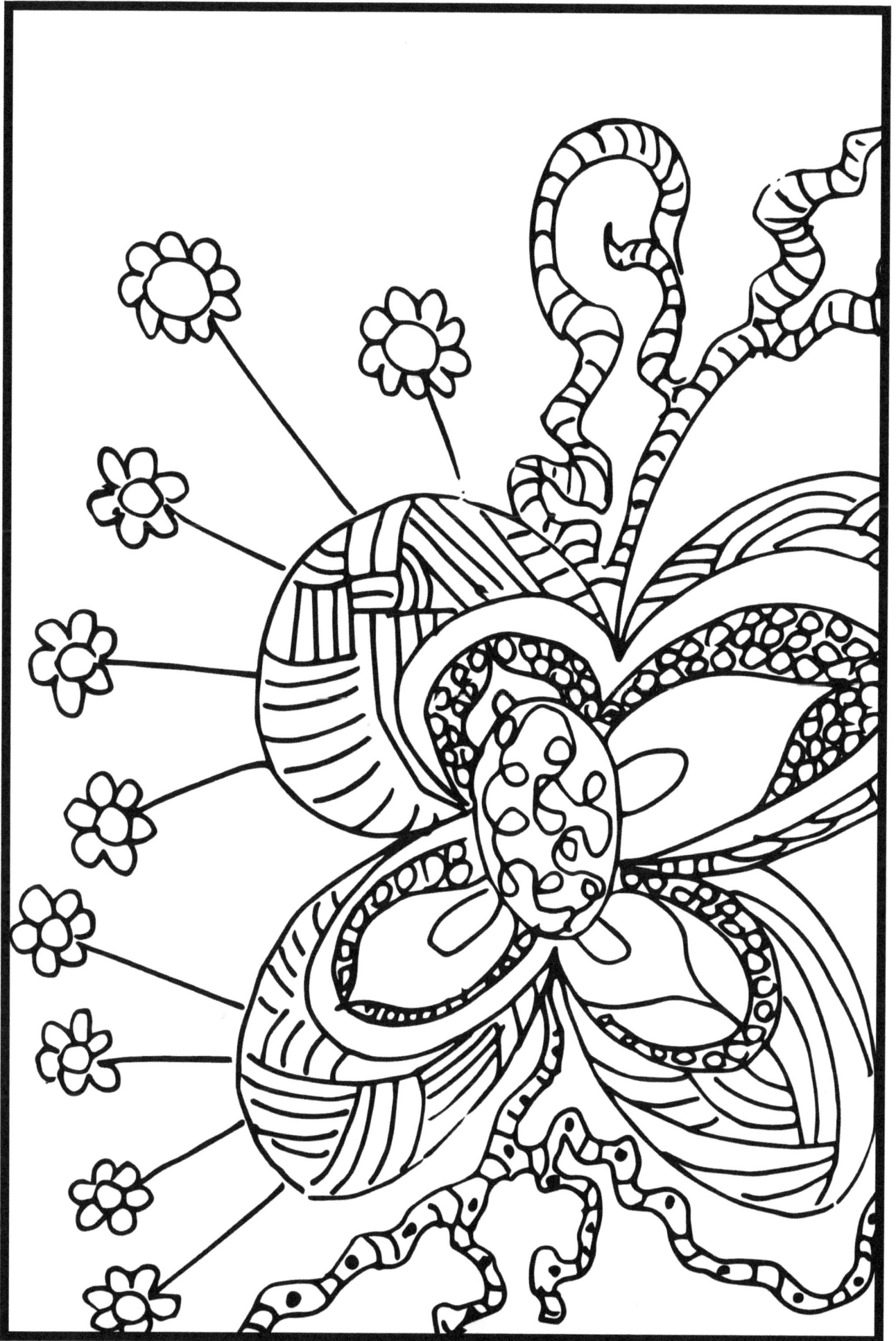

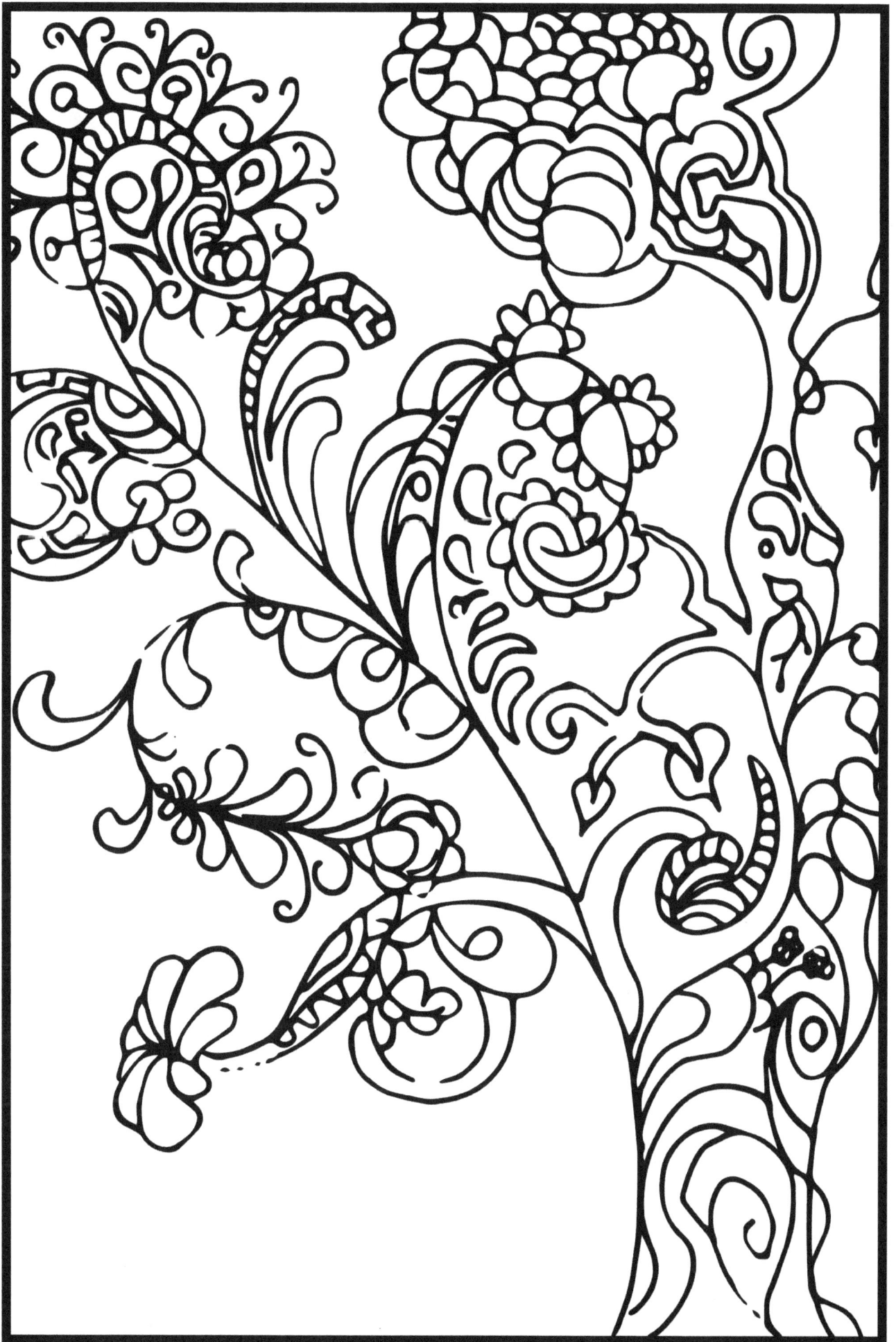

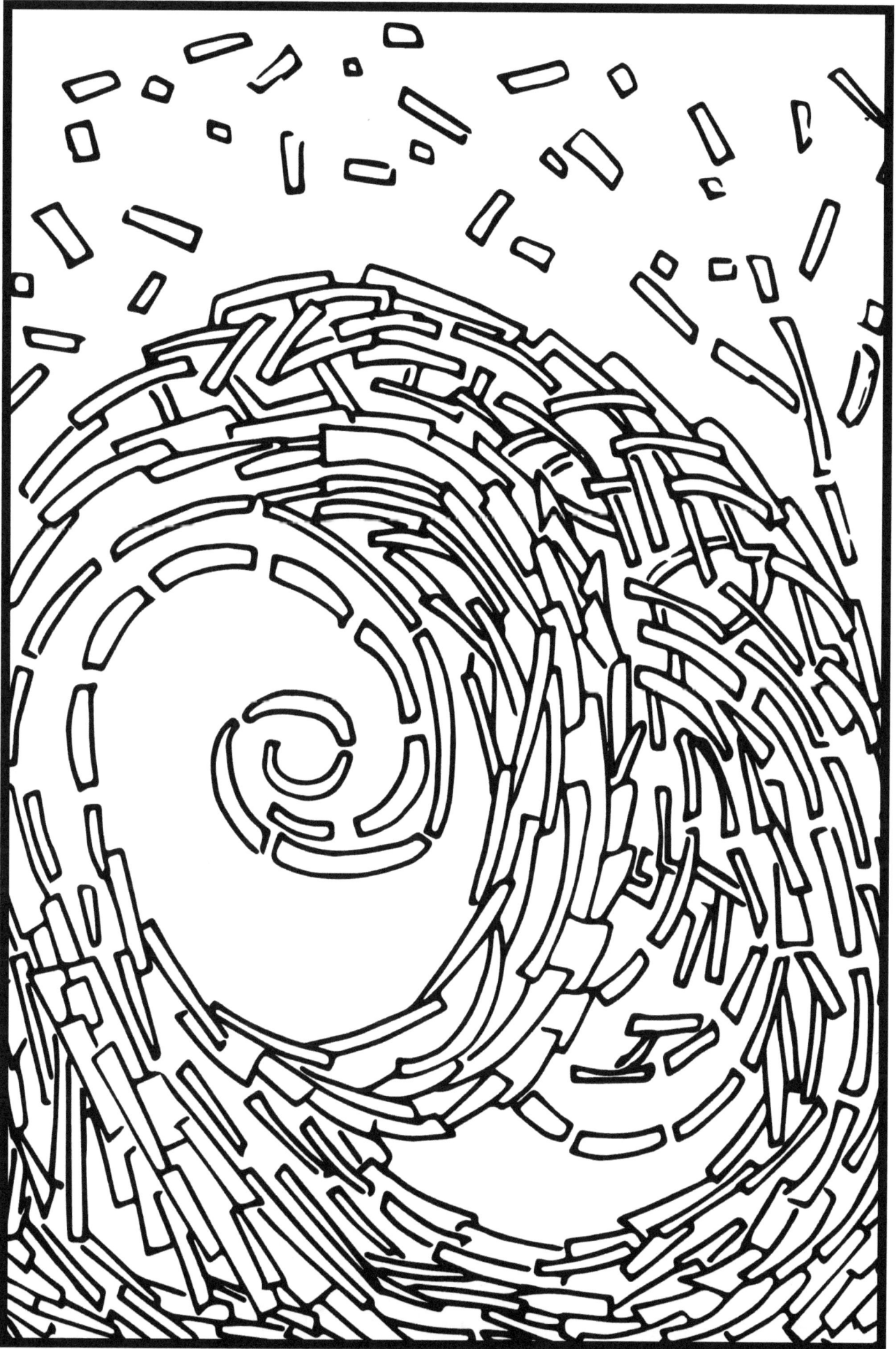

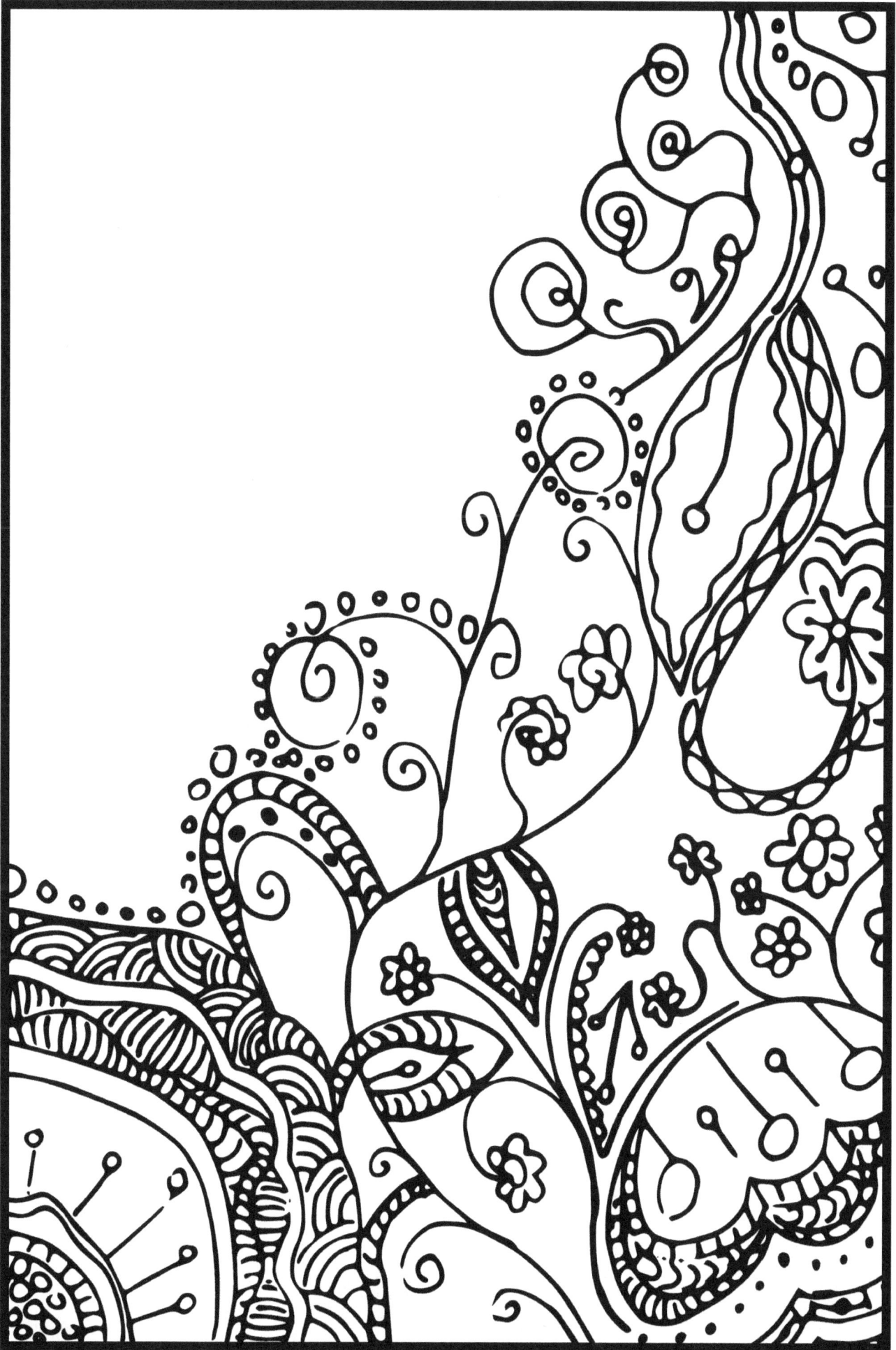

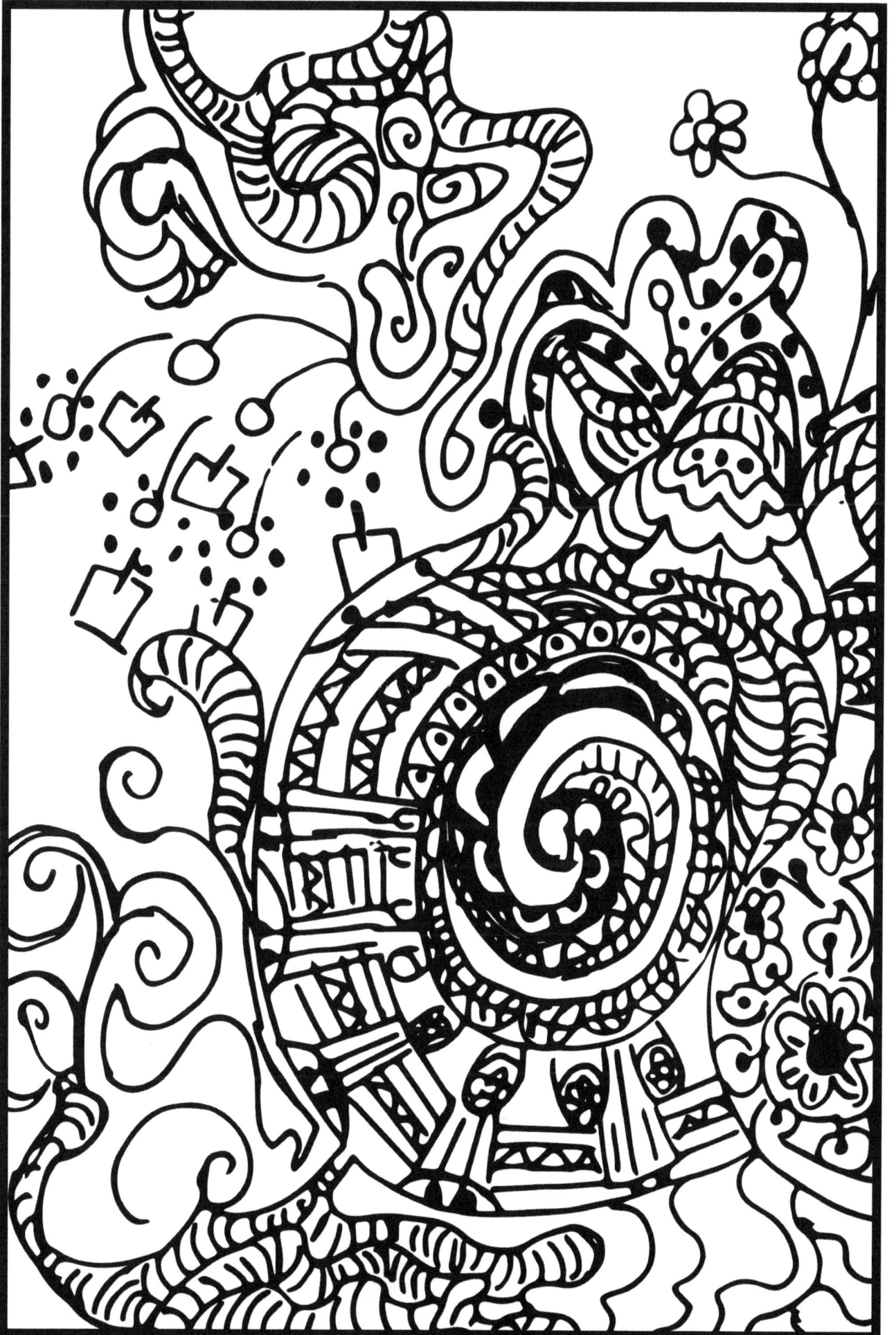

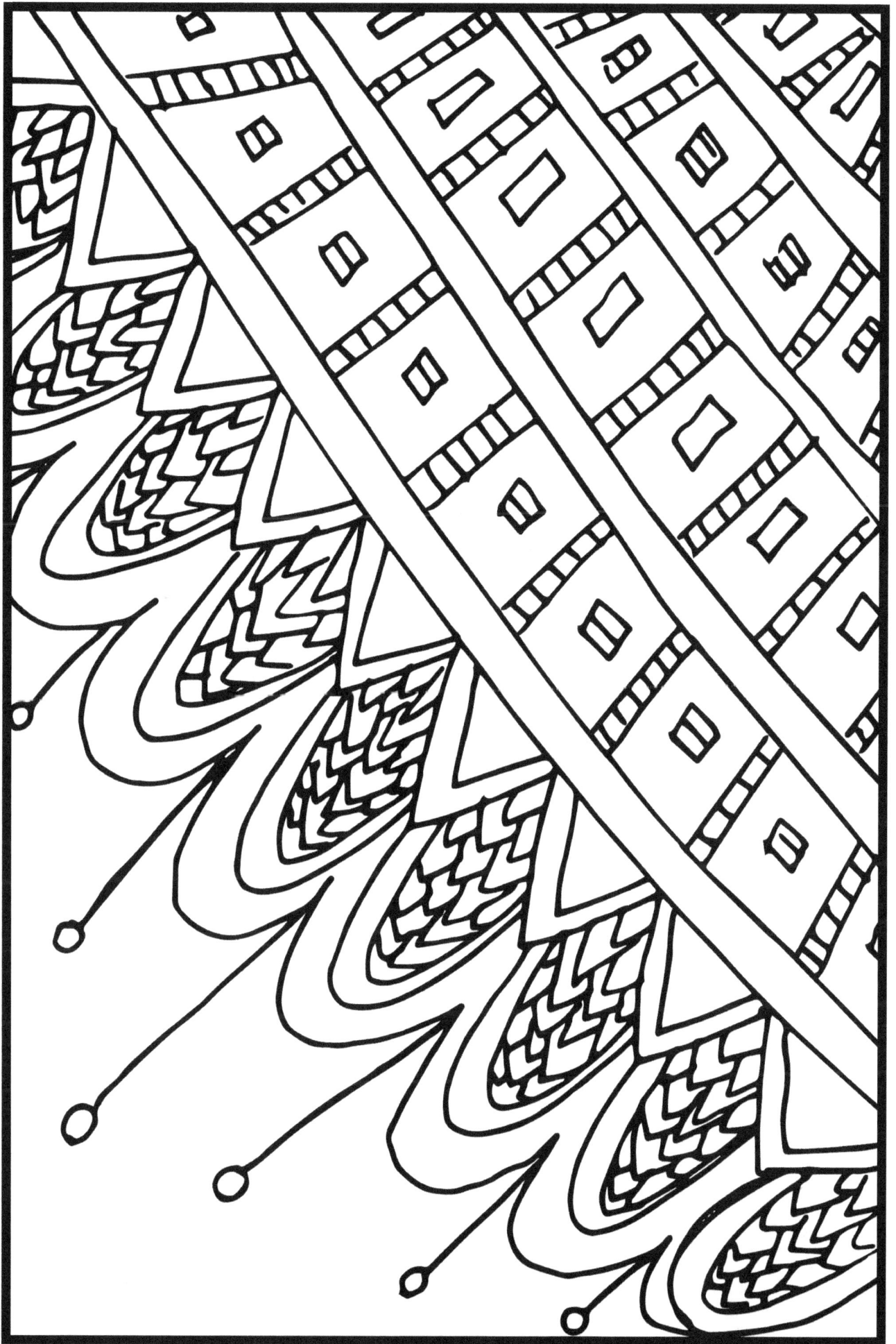

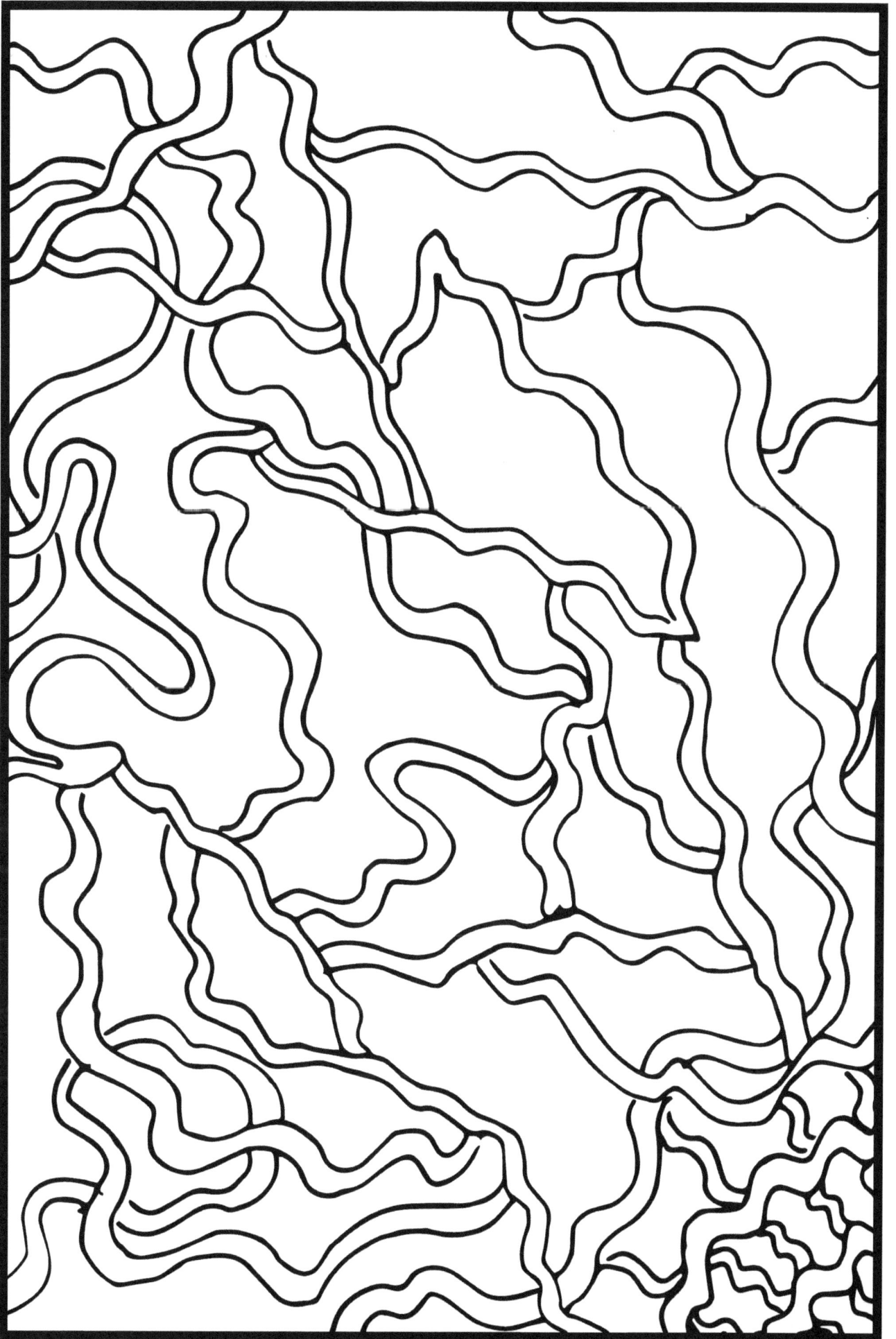

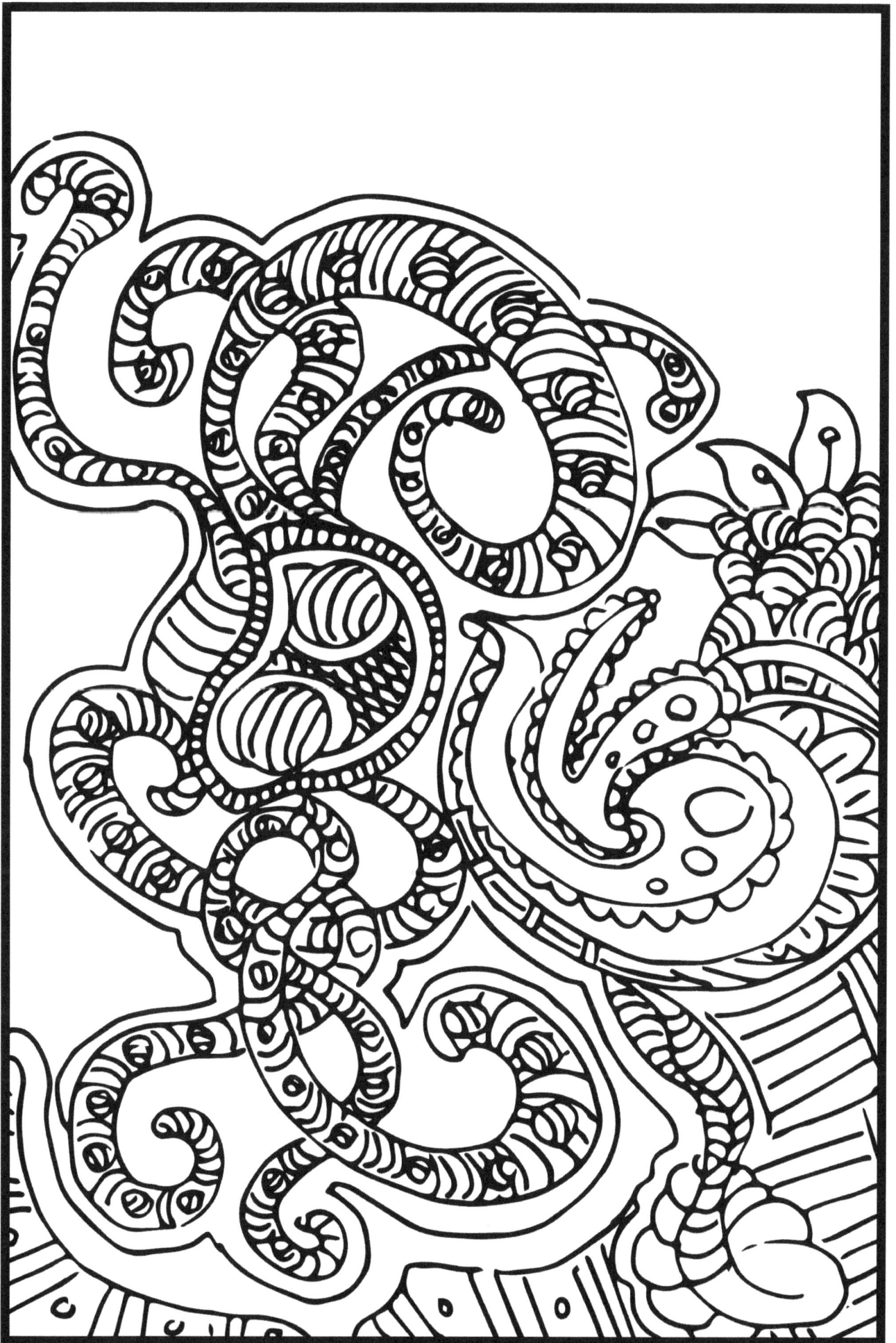

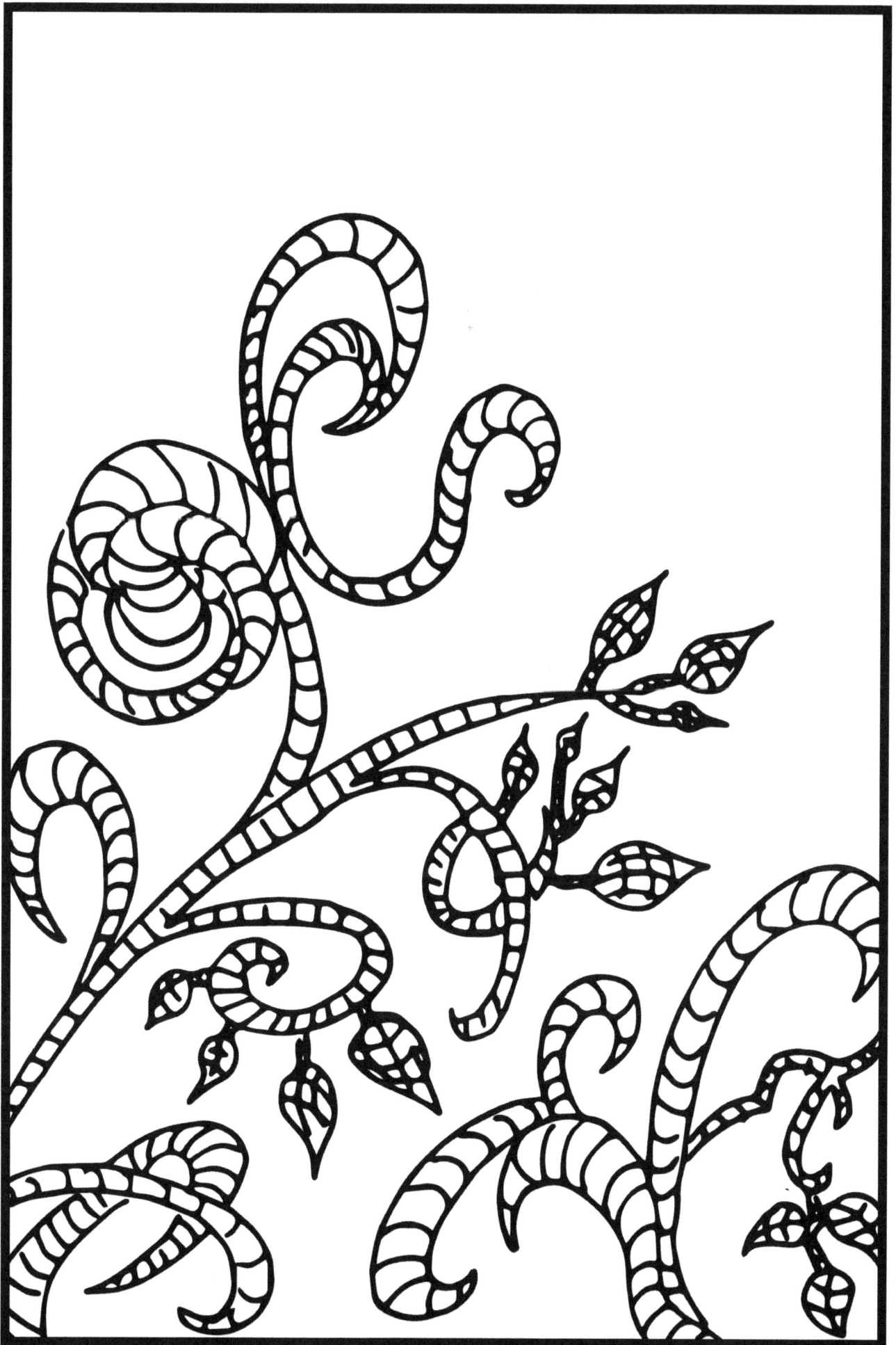

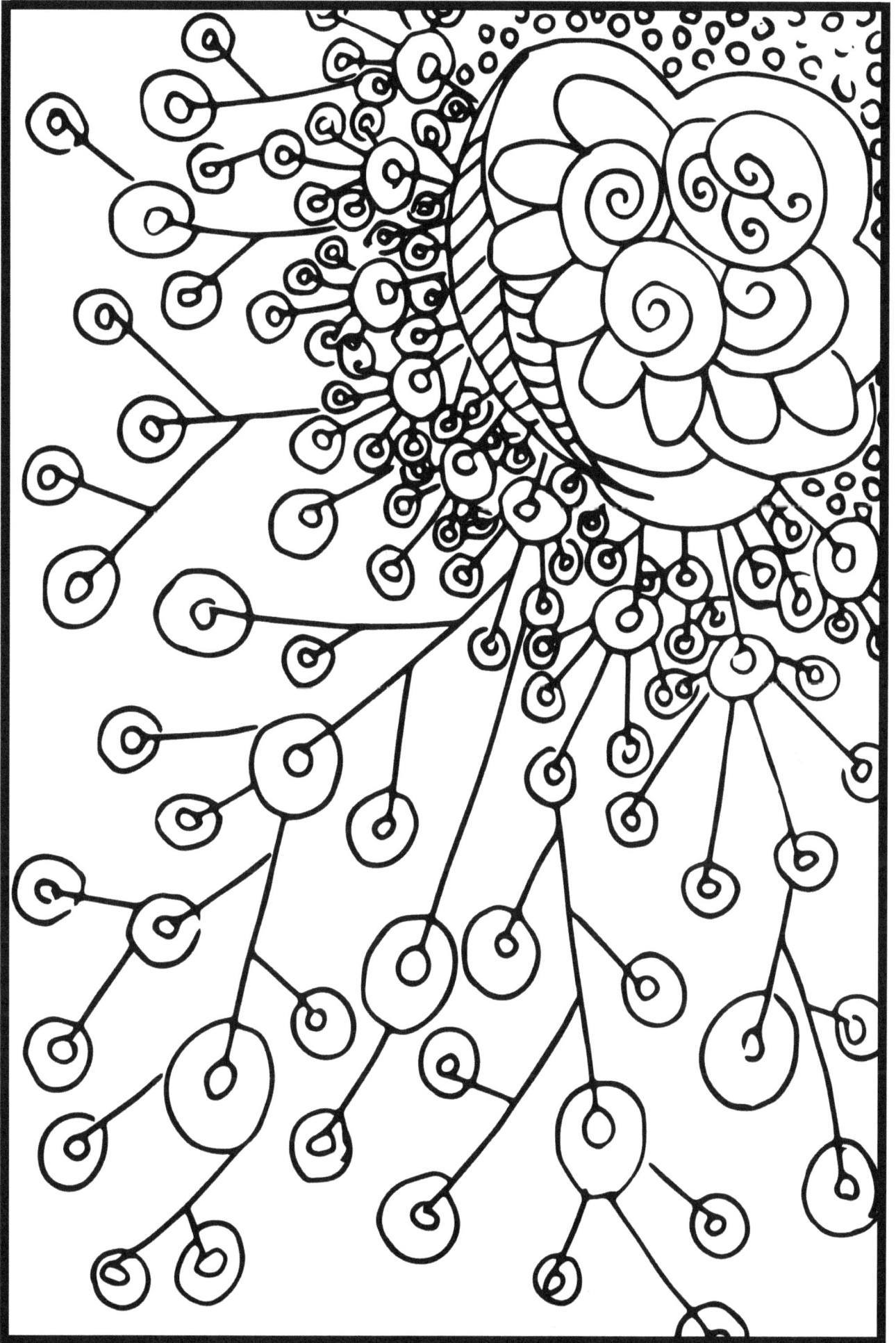

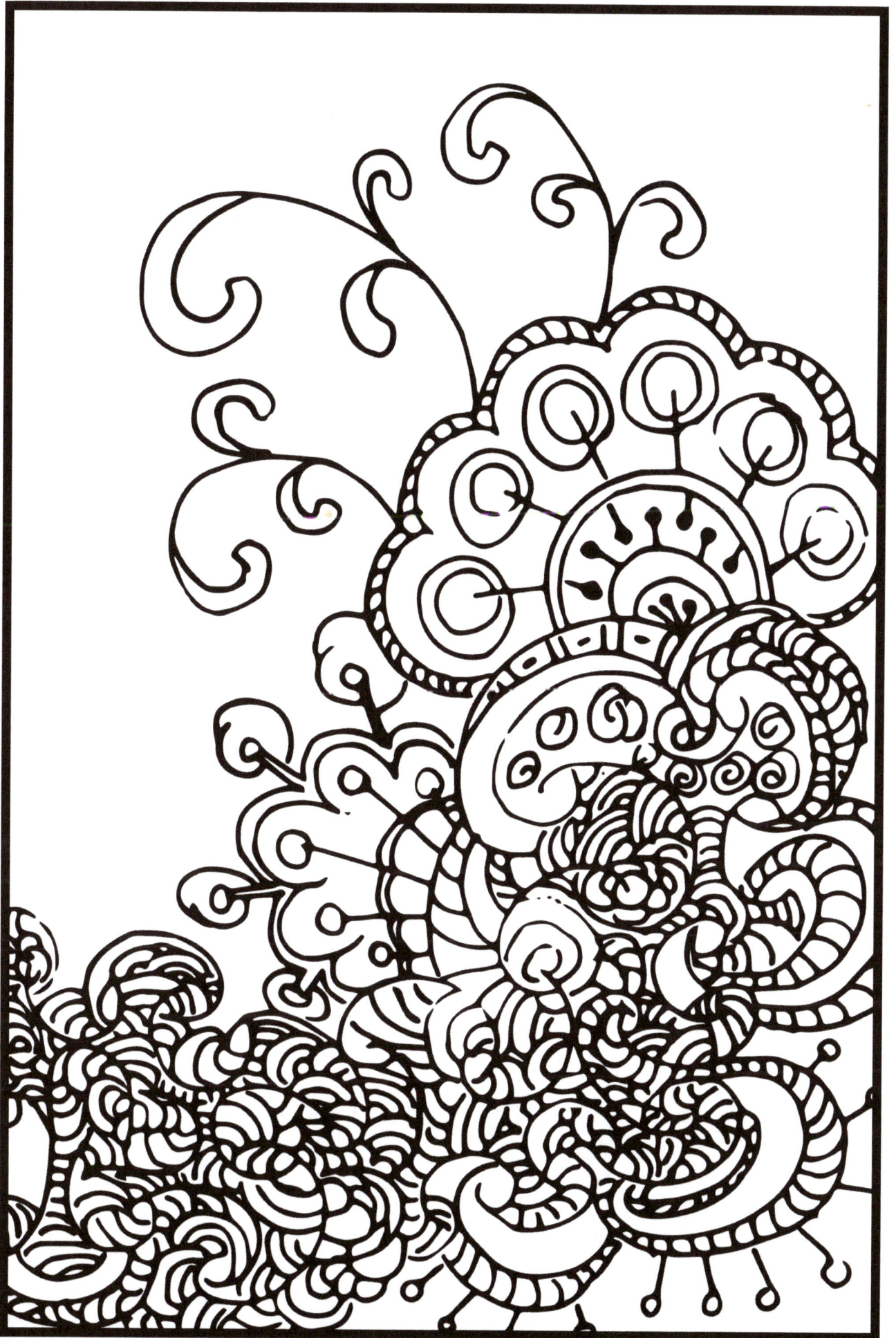

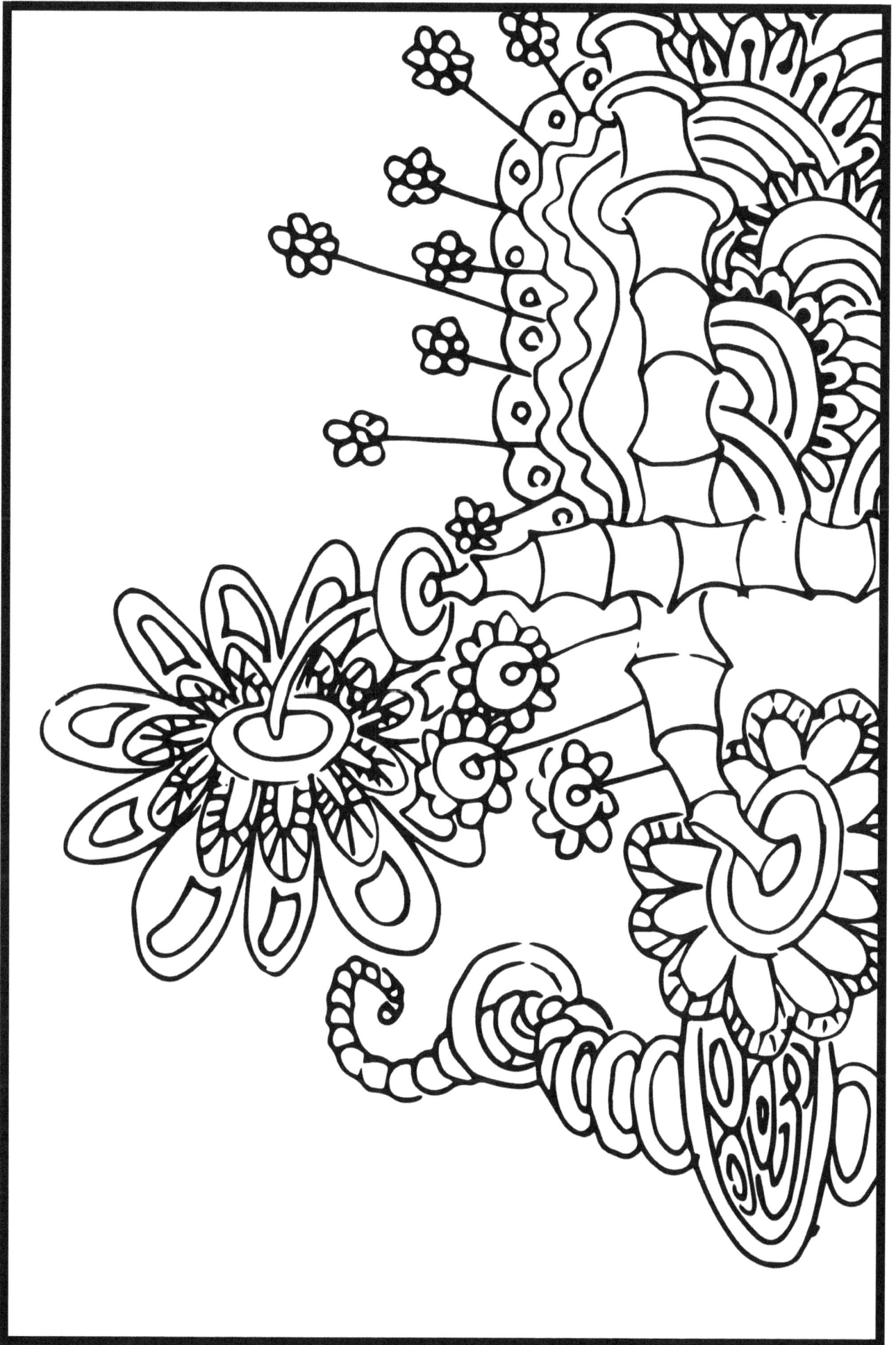

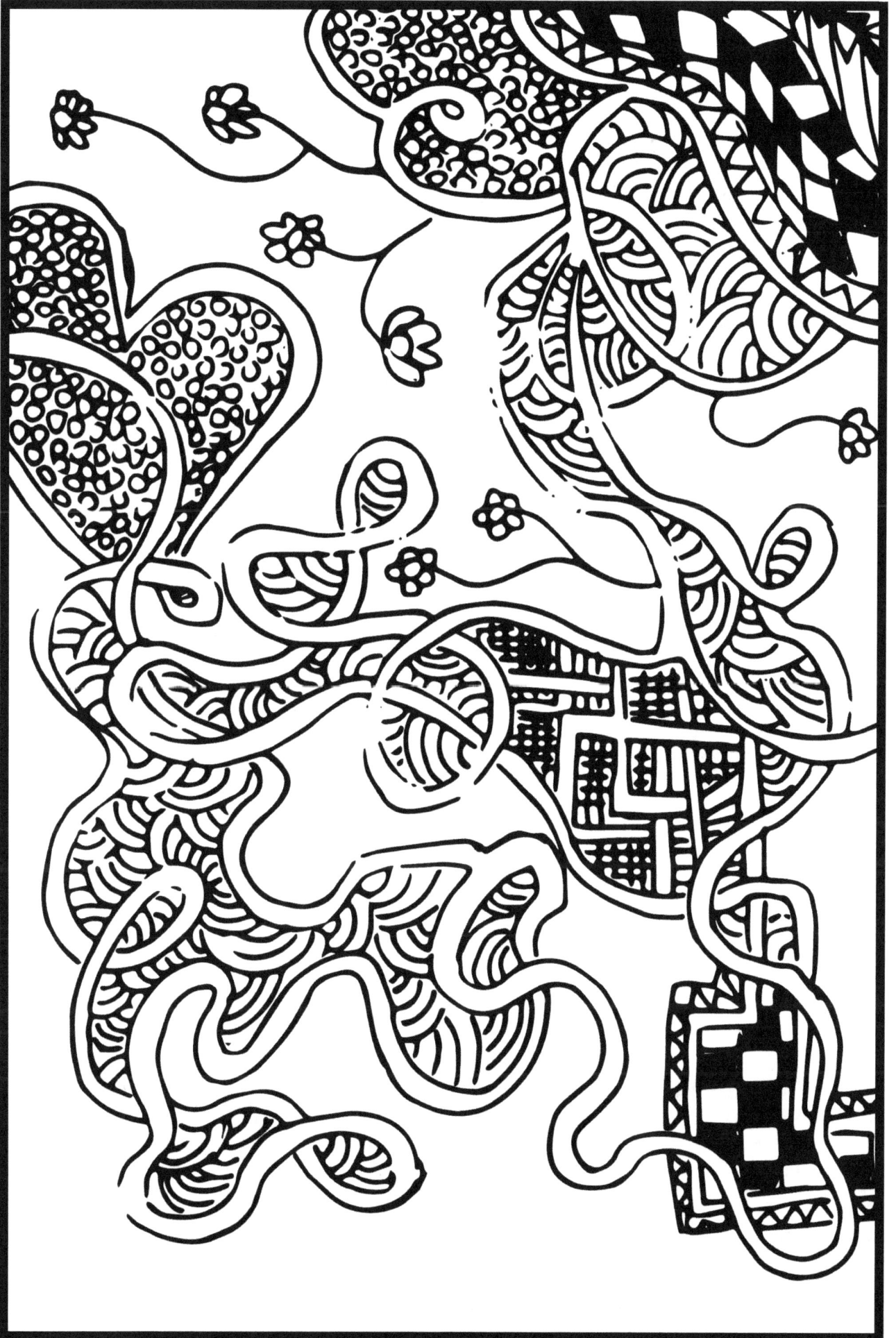

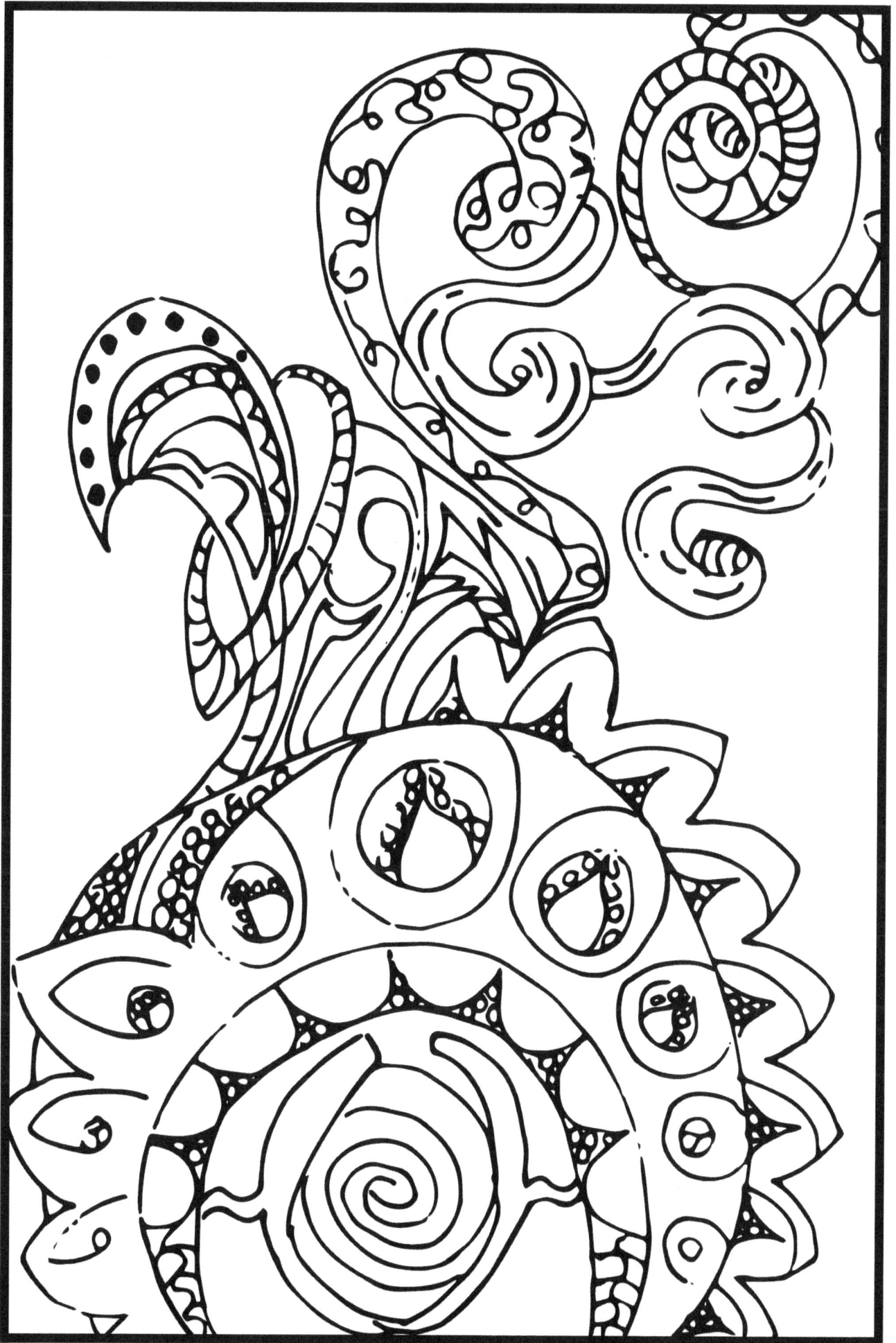

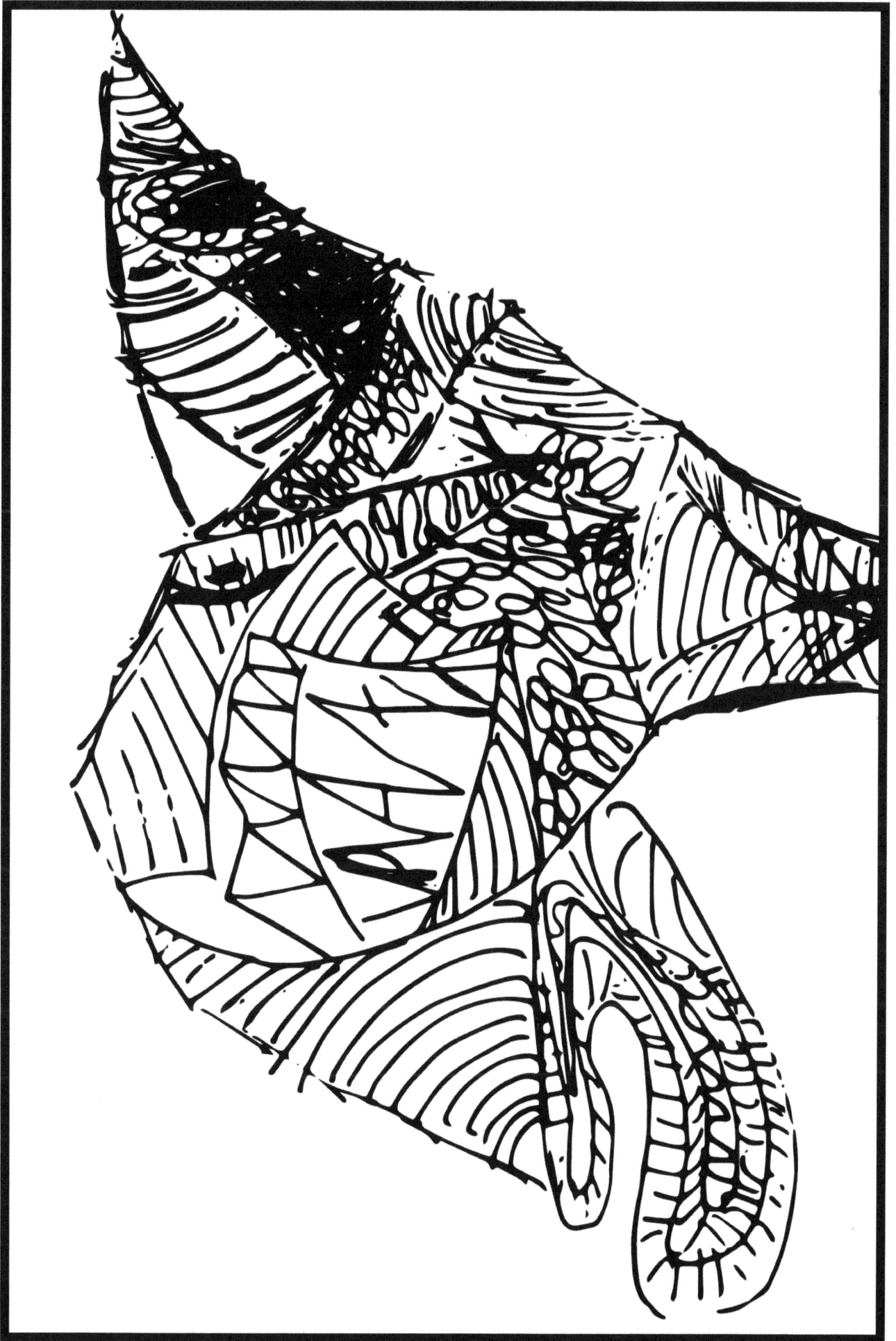

Testing Page!!!
Markers, pencils, oil pastels, or any other medium of your choice here!

Testing Page!!!
Markers, pencils, oil pastels, or any other medium of your choice here!

SASHA SCULLY

Written and Illustrated by Sasha Scully

www.sashascully.com

www.ingramcontent.com/pod-product-compliance
Lightning Source LLC
Chambersburg PA
CBHW081658270326
41933CB00017B/3210